Achilles Heel/ Achilles Tendonitis Explained.

Achilles Tendon Tear, Stretches, Repair, Exercises, Treatments, Recovery, Alternative Therapies, all covered.

by

Robert Rymore

Published by IMB Publishing 2013

Copyright and Trademarks. This publication is Copyright 2013 by IMB Publishing. All products, publications, software and services mentioned and recommended in this publication are protected by trademarks. In such instance, all trademarks & copyright belong to the respective owners. All rights reserved. No part of this book may be reproduced or transferred in any form or by any means, graphic, electronic, or mechanical, including photocopying, recording, taping, or by any information storage retrieval system, without the written permission of the author. Pictures used in this book are either royalty free pictures bought from stock-photo websites or have the source mentioned underneath the picture. Disclaimer and Legal Notice. This product is not legal or medical advice and should not be interpreted in that manner. You need to do your own due-diligence to determine if the content of this product is right for you. The author and the affiliates of this product are not liable for any damages or losses associated with the content in this product. While every attempt has been made to verify the information shared in this publication, neither the author nor the affiliates assume any responsibility for errors, omissions or contrary interpretation of the subject matter herein. Any perceived slights to any specific person(s) or organization(s) are purely unintentional. We have no control over the nature, content and availability of the web sites listed in this book. The inclusion of any web site links does not necessarily imply a recommendation or endorse the views expressed within them. IMB Publishing takes no responsibility for, and will not be liable for, the websites being temporarily unavailable or being removed from the internet. The accuracy and completeness of information provided herein and opinions stated herein are not guaranteed or warranted to produce any particular results, and the advice and strategies, contained herein may not be suitable for every individual. The author shall not be liable for any loss incurred as a consequence of the use and application, directly or indirectly, of any information presented in this work. This publication is designed to provide information in regards to the subject matter covered. The information included in this book has been compiled to give an overview of Achilles tendonitis and detail some of the symptoms, treatments etc. that are available to people with this condition. It is not intended to give medical advice. For a firm diagnosis of your condition, and for a treatment plan suitable for you, you should consult your doctor or consultant. The writer of this book and the publisher are not responsible for any damages or negative consequences following any of the treatments or methods highlighted in this book. Website links are for informational purposes and should not be seen as a personal endorsement; the same applies to the products detailed in this book. The reader should also be aware that although the web links included were correct at the time of writing, they may become out of date in the future.

Table of Contents

Acknowledgements

Special thanks to Dr Nathan Wei from the Arthritis Treatment Center for his help with this book. He is a board certified rheumatologist with more than 30 years of practice and clinical research experience.

Thanks also to physio room for their advice.

Foreword

One of the conditions I see a lot of is Achilles tendinopathy.
The term "tendinopathy" is preferred to the term tendinitis
because, microscopically, there is very little inflammation.
Usually the problem, particularly with patients who go
on to rupture, is wear and tear, hence, the use of the term
"tendinopathy."

Treatment of Achilles tendinopathy involves the use of a lift for the
shoe, rest, and physical therapy. Analgesics may be prescribed for
pain.
Patients who continue to have issues are candidates for ultrasound-
guided needle tenotomy with the injection of platelet-rich plasma
(PRP), which is an ultra concentrate of the patient's own blood.
This ultra concentrate contains a large number of platelets, which
are cells packed with growth and healing factors.

For those unfortunate to have ruptured their Achilles, surgery is
usually required. This is followed by casting and rehabilitation.
Recovery may take up to a year.

Nathan Wei, MD, FACP, FACR, the **Arthritis Treatment
Centre.**

NOTE:

Many doctors now refer to Achilles Tendonitis as Achilles
Tendinopathy. However, as Achilles tendonitis is the name most
people are familiar with, this is the name used in this book, however
the book will also make reference to Achilles tendinopathy.

Introduction

Every year, 1000s of people experience the pain and discomfort of an Achilles problem. This could vary from a mild inflammation of the tendon to a complete rupture. This book focuses largely on Achilles tendonitis, but also highlights some of the other conditions that can affect the Achilles and details treatment options available to people with an Achilles tendon injury. The information in this book will help the reader to find a way forward when it comes to their own personal treatment plan. With all of the various options laid out, it should become easier to find which method of treatment works best for your needs.

As well as being extremely painful, Achilles tendon problems can be incredibly debilitating, and depending on how bad the symptoms get, the pain could start to affect the everyday aspects of your life as well as restrict the types of activities that you enjoy doing. This is why it is so important to find a treatment that is suitable for you and to find out about the many treatment options that are now available for treating Achilles tendonitis, rupture etc.

Dealing with any injury isn't easy – and Achilles tendon pain can be amongst the worst kind of injury for an athlete – but this book should help put you on the right path to finding effective ways of managing the condition and to make your everyday life manageable. This book will explore options from the gentler massage and yoga therapy treatments to surgical options, should they be required.

However, it is not recommended that you try any of the treatment methods detailed in this book without first consulting a doctor, consultant or sports therapist as they are in the best position to assess which treatments would be the most suitable for your particular Achilles problem.

Chapter 1) The Achilles Tendon and Achilles Tendonitis

1) Achilles tendon – History

The term "Achilles Heel" is probably one that you are familiar with, but you may be unaware of its origins.

"Achilles Heel" refers to a person's weak spot. According to Greek mythology, Achilles mother Thetis had a prophecy that her son would die. In order to protect him, she dipped Achilles into the River Styx. However, as his mother lowered Achilles into the water, she held him by the heel, thus this part of Achilles body wasn't protected and it became his vulnerable area.

In the Trojan War, Achilles was struck in the unprotected heel with a poisonous arrow and died as a result.

Some people also refer to the Achilles tendon as the calcaneal tendon. The word "calcaneal" is derived from the Latin word calcaneum, which means heel.

Unfortunately, far too many people will be aware of just how vulnerable this tendon is as they will have experienced an injury to the Achilles at some point.

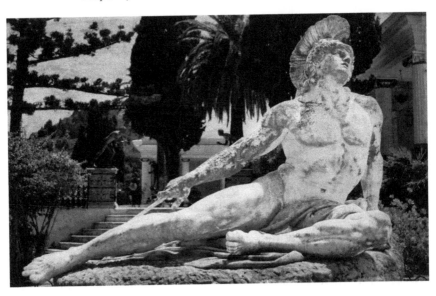

Just as the well-known Greek myth shows, the Achilles tendon can often be the Achilles heel for athletes, leading to both short term and long term damage or injury.

2) About the Achilles tendon

The Achilles tendon is the longest tendon in the human body. The strong, fibrous cords of the Achilles tendon connect the muscles in the calf to the heel bone. While the Achilles tendon is the strongest in the body that does not mean that it is not prone to many injuries including tendonitis and rupture.

The Achilles tendon is vital to the functioning of the foot and for everyday movements. It allows the flexion of the foot and is used in walking, running, jumping, standing on tip toes and climbing the stairs. Day after day, the thick, fibrous cords of the Achilles tendon are called upon to undertake an enormous amount of stress, and sometimes the strain becomes too much for the tendon, which paves the way for inflammation and the degeneration of the Achilles.

14

The tendon is capable of bearing a significant amount of stress; however, this tendon is also prone to overuse injuries and inflammation that can cause on-going pain and discomfort.

People often injure their tendon through repetitive stress or from sudden sharp movements; damage to the Achilles tendon is one of the most common types of sports injury.

While tendons can take a lot of stress, once injured, a tendon can prove difficult to heal; cases of tendonitis can typically take six-eight weeks before it will show signs of improvement. Once healed, it is easy for the tendon to become injured again, especially if you go back to the activities that you were doing before. This book makes some suggestions on how to better manage conditions such as tendonitis, and also offers advice on the many different products that are out there to help patients with this condition

There has also been plenty of new research into treating this Achilles problems, and details of some of the new studies, which offer new hope and insights to people struggling with this painful injury, will be detailed as well.

The other aim of this book is to try and help readers to learn the contributing factors to Achilles tendonitis in order to help avoid this kind of injury.

The hope is to give the reader practical advice so they can learn all they need to know and realise that there are options available for treating their condition.

Armed with the information in this book, you can learn how to manage your Achilles pain effectively, and you can learn what works for you.

From orthotics to yoga postures, this book aims to provide

something for everyone to help ease their Achilles pain.

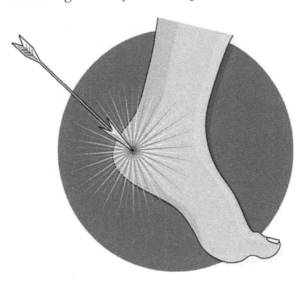

3) Statistics

An Achilles injury is all too common. Syracuse Orthopedic Specialists state that there are more than 250,000 Achilles injuries a year – most of these injuries are sports related.

Out of those suffering an injury, more than 100,000 were unable to partake in sports for a month, while a further 60,000 were still out of action for much longer..

It is estimated that 65,000 people with Achilles tendon injuries had to undergo surgery or therapy.

According to the journal Podiatry Today, Achilles tendonitis is extremely common among athletes; tendonitis accounts for 18% of running injuries and is most common among those competing in long distance running events.

Achilles tendonitis is the third most common injury among athletes, with ankle sprains and plantar fasciitis being the most frequent injuries.

Short term treatment for many patients with this painful condition is often successful, however, in some cases surgery will be considered if there is no other way of alleviating the symptoms. Statistics show that in the cases of surgery there is an 85% success rate, but the surgery is not always successful in the long term and further operations might be needed in the years that follow in order to allow a patient to remain active in their sport.

Surgery carried out on patients with tendonitis, tendinosis, insertional tendonitis and bursitis showed a satisfaction rate of between 67% and 86%. The results for surgery in tendinosis cases showed the poorest results. However, it also needs to be considered that this was just a small group study of just seventy nine people.

4) What is Achilles Tendonitis?

Nathan Wei, MD from the Arthritis Treatment Center explains:

"Achilles tendinopathy is one of the more common forms of tendon disorders.

Predisposing factors for Achilles tendinopathy are abnormal foot motion, excessive weight, prior history of Achilles problems, bad footwear, and a sudden increase in activity.

The most common cause is probably sudden excessive physical training. This increased load leads to inflammation of the tendon sheath as well as degeneration in the tendon.

By far, the most important issue is the tendon degeneration. That is because it is the degeneration that predisposes to rupture.

As the Boomer population remains increasingly active, members of that group will sustain more Achilles injuries. Achilles tendinopathy is painful and limits both the ability to exercise as well as the opportunity to participate in normal day-to-day activities. Even walking is painful.

Early diagnosis and aggressive treatment of Achilles tendinopathy are critical in order to prevent rupture.

The most common "scene" for Achilles rupture is the weekend warrior who goes out to play tennis or basketball without sufficient preparation and stretching. Professional athletes are not immune (Kobe Bryant).

Probably the most exciting development in the treatment of Achilles tendinopathy is the use of ultrasound-guided needle tenotomy with the injection of autologous tissue graft, better known as platelet-rich plasma (PRP).

PRP is an ultra concentrate of blood containing large numbers of platelets, which are cells packed with growth and healing factors.

When carried out by an experienced clinician, the success rate in healing Achilles tendinopathy approaches 95 per cent.

I know about this topic from personal experience since I had an Achilles rupture 31 years ago on my left side treated with surgery and chronic tendinopathy on my right treated with PRP"

5) What causes Achilles tendonitis?

As Dr. Wei explained there are several causes that can contribute to Achilles tendonitis. Other factors that can contribute to this problem include weak or tight calf muscles, diabetes, Reiter's syndrome, doing too much too soon when it comes to exercise, pronation, poorly fitting shoes, soft tissue damage, high arches and flat feet.

This next section will explain in more detail how these issues can contribute to Achilles tendonitis.

Reiter's Syndrome

Reiter's syndrome is a reactionary arthritis. The condition can cause inflammation in the joints as well as the eyes, and can leave the skin vulnerable to lesions. Achilles Tendonitis is also common in people with this syndrome.

Type One Diabetes

Tendonitis is also more common in patients with type one diabetes. Experts are not clear why patients with diabetes are more prone to tendon problems than others. However, there is a theory that an excess of glucose will weaken collagen, thus leading to a weakening of the tendon. The weakness in the tendon will then cause it to become more susceptible to injury.

Ankylosing spondylitis

Also known as Betchterew's syndrome or Marie-Strumpell disease, Ankylosing spondylitis is an inflammation of the axal skeleton. The disease causes symptoms such as pain, swelling, eye pain and fatigue. Ankylosing spondylitis will also contribute to Achilles Tendonitis in some patients.

Age

Problems with the Achilles tendon can also become much more common as we age. With age, the tendon becomes much less flexible and is no longer able to cope with the demands placed on it. It is also not uncommon for people to become "weekend warriors", where they indulge in exercise when they wouldn't do normally and place far too much demand on the tendon than it is used to. This will often result in pain in the Achilles tendon.

Poorly Fitting Shoes

Wearing the right trainers when exercising is vital for giving the feet the support they need when being put under the stress and strain of exercise.

Shoes that don't offer enough support or that don't have enough arch support can leave a person vulnerable to Achilles injury. In addition, if a person is also prone to pronation, they should ideally be wearing custom made orthotics for additional comfort.

High Arched Feet

Having high arches puts an additional strain on the Achilles, as will having flat feet or pronating feet. This can be aided by wearing orthotics and a sports therapist or orthotist will be able to best advise a patient on this.

Tight Calves

Having tight calves can cause stress and irritation to the Achilles tendon, causing pain and inflammation. If this problem is allowed to continue without being treated it can develop into Achilles tendinopathy. You'll find exercises to stretch the calves later on in this book.

Weak Calves

Weak calves will also leave a person prone to Achilles tendonitis. There are exercises in this book designed to help strengthen the calf area, but patients should bear in mind that strong muscles are also tighter, so stretch and strength exercises need to be done together.

Exercising without warming up

Beginning an exercise routine without properly preparing the muscles and tendons for exercise is a sure fire way to contribute to Achilles problems, as well as other sports injuries. Before starting an exercise routine it is important to spend some time stretching and gently warming up the muscles so that they are prepared for exercise. Warming up properly will also increase circulation and blood flow.

Overuse

Everyone knows the feeling they get when they have overused a muscle or tendon. This can often be felt as a burning pain or a limited range of motion in the affected area. Our tendons are only designed to do so much and repeatedly doing the same action will cause an undue burden on the tendon, leading to pain and in some cases, deterioration of the tendon.

However, overuse of the Achilles tendon is avoidable by taking proper precautions such as not exercising without warming up first, wearing supportive trainers and insoles, not doing too much too soon, proper stretching and massage, and by varying workouts to avoid putting too much of the same kind of a stress on a tendon.

Doing Too Much Too Soon

When first starting to exercise, it can be tempting for people to push themselves to their limits and see how far their bodies can go. This is almost guaranteed to end in injury of some sort as the body – including the tendons – simply is not prepared for the extra load they are being asked to endure.

While many people enjoy pushing themselves to their limits, it is not recommended if you are to avoid Achilles injuries.

Biomechanics

A foot that does not work as well as it should will leave a person far more likely to succumb to some sports injuries. As well as Achilles problems, poor biomechanics will leave a person more prone to calf strains, shin splints, ankle pain and ankle sprains.

Dr Nathan Wei explains what biomechanics are and how this can contribute to Achilles tendonitis:

"What this means is that there is a direct correlation between the load applied to the tendon and the amount of strain placed on the tendon. Excessive loading of the tendon during physical activity appears to be the primary culprit responsible for damage.

When excess strain is applied, the tendon fibers undergo microscopic tearing. Repair of this damage is performed by tendon cells. Repetitive stress may not allow the tendon cells to repair the tendon."

"Other factors have been theorized to participate in tendon

damage. These include abnormal free radical damage and the overproduction of destructive cytokines (inflammatory proteins). This latter situation has a clinical model.

Carrying too much weight puts an excessive amount of strain on ligaments and tendons. This can contribute to tendonitis in some patients.

6) Symptoms of Achilles Tendonitis

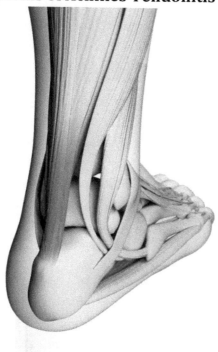

The symptoms of tendonitis often come on slowly. Often so slowly that the patient might not always realise that there is a problem until the symptoms become more severe and more difficult to treat. Symptoms will usually begin with a pain at the bottom of the calf and can sometimes be felt either side of the tendon. Patients might also notice that the pain is worse in the morning and there might also be some stiffness, too. The pain can also be felt during and after exercise and if left untreated a patient can reach the point where the pain becomes a constant part of their lives.

Patients with Achilles tendonitis will also feel pain during activity that requires weight bearing on the affected foot. Climbing the stairs will also trigger pain in some patients and putting weight through the affected heel can become difficult.

Other symptoms of Achilles tendonitis include tenderness around the Achilles area, redness, a thickening of the tendon and pain in the ankle.

If the tendon goes untreated then the patient might notice that the tendon begins to thicken and swell. This can make wearing shoes difficult and can change the way that a patient walks, which in turn can add more stress to the tendon. If the swelling continues it can also reach the point where the tendon swells into the back of the ankle, leaving the ankle joint looking disfigured. However, this is only in severe cases that have been left untreated, which is why early treatment and detection of this condition is so important.

7) Diagnosis of Achilles Tendonitis

Your doctor won't usually need to send you for any tests to establish that you have Achilles tendonitis. The symptoms of this condition are pretty telling and if you have pain in the Achilles area, the Achilles looks inflamed, swollen or feels tender to the touch, and if there is additional swelling in the ankle, your GP will probably suspect tendonitis.

Your GP should also check for any other areas of tenderness in case it is indicative of any other injury. Your GP might also ask questions about what you were doing before the injury to help establish what has happened, and your GP might check the range of motion.

During the initial examination you might also be asked to stand so that your doctor can view your Achilles and they might also look for signs of pronation or biomechanical problems. If your doctor notices any problems with your gait that could be contributing to your tendon pain, then you might be referred to an orthotist. An orthotist will be able to make suggestions of suitable orthotics, and these are available on the NHS.

If the pain is severe then you might be sent for an x-ray to rule out a fracture or a stress fracture. A scan won't normally be necessary to confirm your diagnosis and scans can often be difficult to obtain via the NHS. If you are concerned over the damage that might have been caused to a tendon and you want a clearer idea of what is going on then you might want to ask for a referral to go for a scan privately.

Going for a scan isn't as expensive as some people might think, and your GP can make this referral for you. Charges usually start at £180.00 and you can then go back to your own doctor for the results if you don't want the expense of follow up appointments.

There are two different types of scans. The first is an ultrasound scan than will help to determine any damage done to the tendon. There is also the option of an MRI scan, and this will produce the most detailed picture.

If your doctor is concerned that you might have ruptured your Achilles tendon then they will test this by asking you to lie flat on your stomach while they bend your knee up towards you. If you have ruptured your tendon then your foot will either have to be casted or you'll have to consider Achilles surgery to repair the damage that has been done.

You'll find a chapter on Achilles ruptures later on in this book and you'll also discover the treatment options currently available.

8) Surgery for Tendonitis

In rare cases – and when all other treatment options have proved ineffective – your consultant might suggest surgery to repair the damaged tendon. However, surgery won't normally be considered unless your tendonitis has continued for six months or more.

Unfortunately, surgery is not guaranteed to cure your Achilles tendonitis and you could still experience on-going pain. There is also a limited chance of complications such as developing an infection or a blood clot due to inactivity.

The American Academy of Orthopedic Surgeons detail three options for Achilles repair.

Gastrocnemius Recession

During this type of surgery the calf will be lengthened. Excessively tight calves cause stress to the Achilles so lengthening the calf should prevent this from happening.

The lengthening of the calf will also increase the range of motion in the ankle.

The surgery is carried out by using a traditional incision or by using an endoscopic incision.

Debridement

During a tendon debridement, a surgeon will remove the injured part of the tendon. Once the damaged part of the tendon has been removed, the surgeon will then stich the Achilles. If you suffer from insertional Achilles tendonitis then the surgeon will also remove the heel spur. Recovery time from this kind of surgery is typically two weeks and you might be told to wear a walking cast while the tendon heels.

Debridement with tendon transfer

This type of surgery will be an option when the Achilles has been more than 50% damaged. If 50% of the tendon is removed, that means there simply isn't enough healthy tendon left for it to be able to function well. This would leave the patient vulnerable to complications such as Achilles rupture.

In cases such as this, a tendon transfer will also need to be carried out to replace the damaged tendon.

Although the results from this surgery are mainly good, recovery time is lengthy – up to twelve months. A minority of patients will also continue to feel pain after the surgery.

9) Treatment of Achilles Tendonitis/Tendinopathy

Tendonitis is best treated sooner than later as it is easier to treat in its early stages. On the first onset of pain, it is important to rest rather than try and push through the pain and risk making the pain worse.

Anti-inflammatory

Although many medical practitioners now believe the cause of most tendon problems is the degeneration of the tendon, in the early stages of the pain and swelling, doctors will still advocate taking an anti-inflammatory such as ibuprofen as it may be effective at reducing these symptoms. These are available over the counter and usually come in 200mg doses. However, if the patient visits their doctor then they might be prescribed anti-inflammatory at a higher dose of 400mg to see if this will help counter the pain and inflammation caused by the early stages of tendonitis.

Precautions:

NSAIDs are generally considered safe; however, people with stomach problems should be careful when taking this type of medication. If you have been prescribed this type of medication on a long term basis, then it is important that a doctor monitors that the NSAIDs aren't causing any long term side effects. It also should be borne in mind that some studies have shown the NSAIDs might inhibit the tendon from healing.

Painkillers

Your doctor might also prescribe paracetamol or a medication containing both paracetamol and codeine such as diclofenac to help reduce the pain. The patient might also be prescribed other medications such as Naproxen if other forms of anti-inflammatory don't prove effective.

Corticosteroids

Although many doctors now accept the problems caused to the Achilles tendon aren't all down to inflammation, the first line of action of many doctors is to prescribe an anti-inflammatory.

If anti-inflammatory medications don't prove effective at combating the pain, it might be suggested that the patient is given a series of corticosteroid injections. Corticosteroids help to reduce inflammation and can be given in tablet or injection form. When it comes to treating cases of Achilles Tendonitis, corticosteroid injections are often used. However, these can cause other side effects such as dizziness, nausea and headaches; in some cases it is thought that corticosteroids can weaken tendons and cause a rupture.

Corticosteroids are not suitable for long term use and diabetics need to be particularly careful of this form of treatment as the injections can cause elevated blood sugar levels.

Rest

The patient will also be advised to rest the injured leg as much as possible and perhaps sit with the foot elevated to help reduce any swelling in the lower limb. Icing the tendon will also be suggested. The best way to do this is to use either an ice pack of a bag of frozen vegetables, wrap it in a towel to avoid the ice coming in direct contact with the skin to prevent ice burns or frostbite or tissue injury. Ice should only be used against the injured tendon for a maximum of 20 minutes, less if you have any kind of circulation problems.

Some patients find that ice doesn't work so well for them and find that heat works better as it can help to relax the muscles. It is just a matter of finding out which methods works best for you.

Ultrasound

Ultrasound therapy is often used to help treat tendonitis. Ultrasound works by increasing the heat to the injured area and speeding up healing. Ultrasound works better for some patients than it does for others; it all depends on how an individual responds to this type of treatment. Ultrasound treatments are usually carried out for up to five minutes at a time. This kind of treatment is usually carried out by a physiotherapist and is available from most private sport injury clinics.

Sports Taping

Taping the ankle to give the joint more support can take some of the pull of the tendons. Sports taping can help take the strain off a tendon while it heals and taping works particularly well with people who participate in a lot of sport and find that it puts a lot of stress on the Achilles tendon. A sports therapist will be able to strap the foot and demonstrate the best way to tape the foot ahead of any events the patient might be taking part in.

Sports taping can also be used to help combat some of the biomechanical problems a patient might have, but it is no means a cure. For instance, if a patient's foot pronates, putting a lot of stress on the Achilles tendon, then strapping the foot to help control the pronation can help. However, strapping isn't suitable for everyone and patients should take special care if they have circulation problems. Patients shouldn't attempt to strap their foot themselves and should seek expert advice instead.

Physiotherapy

A physiotherapist can work with a patient to help find the best treatment for them. This may involve sports massage and stretching techniques, which should focus on stretching the Achilles tendon, calf and soleus muscle. Patients might also be given ankle stretches. Strengthening exercises might also be introduced once the initial pain has subsided and once the patient is able to resume exercise without causing any further pain.

Biomechanics

If the cause of the problem is biomechanical, then the patient will likely be advised to wear inserts or insoles to help control problems like pronation. The Achilles typically takes 6-8 weeks to heal and once it does, patients should take care not to do too much too soon and to make sure that they do a proper warm up and cool down to reduce their risk of re-injury. Patients should also integrate a regular stretch programme into their workouts to ensure that the tendon does not become too tight and prone to inflammation.

iHeal

The iHeal Tissue and Cell Repair Unit is designed to work on soft tissue injuries including tendonitis. The unit uses pulsed electromagnetic fields to help accelerate the time taken for an injury to heal. It is claimed to make the healing process 30% faster and is compact enough for a patient to carry with them for use when they need it.

However, this type of therapy is not right for everyone; it should not be used if you are pregnant, for patients with a heart condition or for people with a pacemaker. The iHeal should also not be used on children aged under 16 years.

TENS

Transcutaneous Electrical Nerve Stimulation is a preferred method of pain relief for many people. TENS machines are used for both acute and chronic pain and they are generally considered safe to use. The TENS machine is attached to the skin via electrodes that send electrical signals to nerves and help combat pain.

The evidence on just how effective TENS machines are is mixed and there are plenty of mixed reviews about the effectiveness of TENS, however, it clearly works for some people and is a good alternative for those that don't want to take painkillers or depend on other kinds of medication.

Before using a TENS machine it is best to consult a doctor as they are not suitable for everyone and should not be used by patients with a heart condition.

Anti-inflammatory gels

Anti-inflammatory gels are ideal for massaging gently into the sore spots of the Achilles pain. They can be used to help reduce the pain and swelling associated with an inflamed tendon, but if the patient has stomach problems then they should be careful about how often they use NSAIDS. These types of gels should not be used over long periods and if the symptoms continue then medical advice should be sought.

Glucosamine Patches

Glucosamine patches are more effective on joint pain; however, if a patient has developed ankle pain due to the Achilles tendonitis then these patches can be useful in helping to reduce the pain. They tend to have a cooling effect, and this in itself can take away some of the discomfort, especially if the ankle joint has become inflamed and the pain feels like it is burning.

Lidocaine Patches

If other attempts to reduce pain have failed then Lidocaine patches are also available to help manage the discomfort. These patches are readily available in the United States and are often used for the treatment of tendonitis. They can cause skin irritation in some patients, but otherwise they seem to be safe overall.

Patients should not attempt to use these patches without first taking advice from their doctor or consultant.

Platelet Rich Plasma

One new treatment that has gotten a lot of attention in recent years is Platelet Rich Plasma therapy or PRP. The treatment involves injecting platelet-rich plasma into the affected tendon over a period of weeks.

PLP has been shown to be effective in cases of Achilles tendonitis, retrocalcaneal bursitis, plantar fasciitis, Achilles heel pain, and tendon pain.

The use of PRP can improve healing time and help to reduce pain while the tendon heals, however, it won't work for everyone and depending on where you live, the treatment might not be available on the NHS..

Who is more likely to suffer an Achilles injury?

A recent study by the American Orthopedic Foot and Ankle Society showed that male athletes are more likely to suffer from an Achilles rupture. The sport most likely to cause this type of injury was basketball.

As part of the study, three doctors - Drs. Steven Raikin, David Garras and Philip Krapchev - reviewed a decade's worth of records and examined the cases of more than 400 patients. The statistics from the study showed that the average age for an Achilles rupture was 46; 83% of people with this injury were men, and 68% of them were playing sport at the time of their injuries.

While basketball caused the most Achilles injuries, sports such as tennis and football were also common causes of tendon injury.

Older people and people with a high Body Mass Index were more likely to have this injury due to non- sports related activity, and a third of injuries were caused at work.

The study also showed that some patients were mistakenly told that they had sprained an ankle, which delayed medical treatment.

5% of the patients had experienced a re-rupturing of the tendon, while 6% had previously ruptured the other tendon.

The Doctors behind the study also made it clear that early treatment is essential in the case of an Achilles rupture, as those who don't have their injury diagnosed or treated in a timely fashion will find themselves taking a much longer time to recover.

The doctors also advised that elderly people and those with a high Body Mass Index should be monitored carefully if they present with swelling in the Achilles area as this could be a sign of a rupture.

Women and Achilles Tendonitis

Although studies show that Achilles ruptures are more common in men, there are many factors that can leave a woman vulnerable to Achilles problems such as tendonitis.

High Heels

First of all, wearing high heels can cause the Achilles to shorten, making it difficult to place the heel on the ground even when not wearing heels. Having the foot placed in the plantar flexed position all day can also contribute to Achilles tendonitis, due to the un-natural position of the foot. Women who wear high heels and then change to flat shoes or trainers are also more prone to this condition as the foot will suddenly need to adapt to walking in a flat position that it isn't used to.

If you absolutely must wear high heels, try a branded insole like Insolia. These have been designed to take the pressure off a woman's foot while they are wearing heels, and they have a slim line design so they will fit into heels.

A study published in 2012 by the Neuromuscular Research Centre, Department of Biology of Physical Activity, University of Jyväskylä, Finland, showed that the long term use of high heels caused the medial gastrocnemius muscle fascicles to shorten as well as causing stiffness in the Achilles.

And the problems high heels can cause to women's feet don't end there. A study published by Houston Medicine showed that of the 39% of women that wear heels every day, 75% of them suffered from bunions, calluses, hammer toes, arthritis in the big toe and plantar warts. The study author also pointed out that due to the shortening of the calf muscles caused by wearing heels this can also cause Achilles tendonitis, plantar fasciitis and flat feet – another contributor to Achilles tendon problems.

Pregnancy

Increased weight and fluid round the feet and ankles can cause women to be more prone to foot problems. The body will also release hormones that help the muscles to relax during pregnancy, however, these hormones can also cause the foot to weaken, meaning that there can be a tendency towards foot pain and injury.

Periods

If you've ever thought that your period can make the pain of your Achilles injury worse, then you are right. Hormones change pain responses and also affect pain management. Moreover, in the days before your period, cortisol levels surge; cortisol can trigger inflammation, leaving you more vulnerable to pain.

Fallen Arches

Fallen arches will leave a woman more prone to Achilles tendonitis as well as a condition called Posterior tibial tendon dysfunction. It is thought that changes in hormones – especially during the menopause – can cause collagen to weaken.

Age

A study published online in Biomedcentral.com showed that older women who were at the post-menopausal or pre-menopausal stage were more likely to have abnormal Achilles tendons.

The study also showed that women with less body fat were also more likely to have an abnormal Achilles tendon.

Hormones

Another study published by FootLogic indicated that women on estrogen therapy or oral contraceptives have a higher prevalence of Achilles tendinopathy. A contributing factor to this is the fact that an increase in estrogen can reduce the levels of collagen, hence weakening the tendon and leaving it exposed to injury.

Casual Footwear

Some types of casual footwear will put an additional strain on the Achilles tendon and will contribute to conditions such as Achilles tendonitis. Because of the way some shoes are designed, they can make the Achilles sore by adding too much pressure to the back of the foot.

Trainers that offer some support would be better than wearing a shoe that is too close to the ground and doesn't offer much protection to the foot.

When choosing trainers, you need to check that they offer enough room at the toe box, that they have a supportive arch, and that your foot can fit comfortably in them. Don't be tempted to jam your foot into trainers that are uncomfortable for your feet.

Fashion

Many women feel like they have to keep up with the latest fashions, but when it comes to footwear, trying to keep up with the latest trends can play havoc with your feet – especially your Achilles tendon.

Some women are not designed to wear high heels or the latest pair of designer shoes. It is important to go with what is comfortable for you and not choose something that might give you a short period of pleasure, but then cause you long term pain.

Get into the habit of wearing what is comfortable for you and wearing something that suits your type of foot. If Achilles pain is a problem for you, then don't make it worse by trying to force an already sore foot into shoes that won't support you when you walk.

Wearing proper footwear can go a long way towards preventing the painful condition of tendonitis, and can help prevent other types of foot problems as well.

Chapter 2) Other Types Of Achilles Tendon problems.

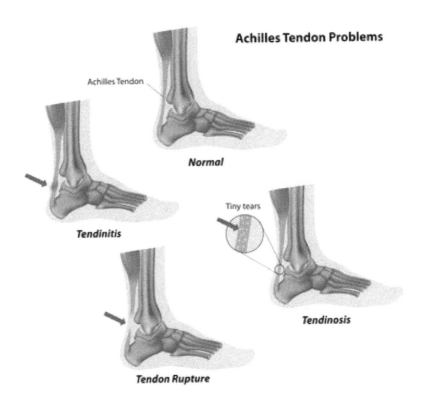

Achilles Tendon Problems

1) Achilles Tendon Rupture

The one injury most athletes dread is the Achilles Rupture. This painful injury led to England star David Beckham missing out on his dream of playing in a fourth World Cup when in 2010 his Achilles ruptured while playing for AC Milan. Beckham left the pitch in tears and had to undergo surgery to repair the damaged tendon

An Achilles tendon can be prone to rupture when an excessive

38

amount of stress or strain is put on it. Any movements that suddenly impact the foot or ankle area can cause a rupture, and it is a common running injury in sports that require lots of push off such as basketball.

This type of injury also takes a long time to recover from and it is possible that the tendon could be ruptured again.

Although this injury is most common in sports stars, it can also occur when your ankle is forced into sudden dorsiflexion or plantar flexion and some medications can also make a person more prone to an Achilles rupture. A rupture can also be caused by a trip or a fall.

Here are some of the other common factors in the causes of Achilles rupture:

- Achilles tendonitis

- Cortisone injections

- Some medications

- Your age

- Changes in your exercise routine

- New activity

Achilles tendonitis can increase your risk of an Achilles rupture as tendonitis will weaken the tendon, leaving it more vulnerable to this type of injury. However, most doctors will advise you that the risk of a rupture developing from tendonitis is small.

Cortisone injections are often given during the first stages of treatment of tendonitis, but some doctors prefer not to use cortisone as it could increase the risk of a rupture.

Certain types of medications can also increase the chances of a tendon rupturing, although these risks will be small. Some antibiotics have been known to cause a rupture. The potential side effects should always be listed and if your medication has been associated with Achilles ruptures, then it will say so in the information leaflet included in the packet. If you are concerned about the medication you have been prescribed, don't stop taking your medication, but do seek advice from your doctor.

Age is another factor in Achilles rupture. As we age, the tendons become less flexible and a sudden, sharp move could be all that is needed to cause an injury. Tendons also take longer to heal as we age.

A sudden change in the amount of sports training done or trying a new activity can also make a tendon more likely to rupture. If you suddenly intensify your training programme it can cause the tendon to work far harder than it normally would, causing injury. New activity will give your muscles and tendons a challenge they are not used to, and this sudden change in what is required of your tendons can leave a person more susceptible to this kind of injury.

2) Symptoms of an Achilles Rupture

Many people who have experienced a rupture will say that it feels like a sharp kick or stabbing pain in the back of the leg. The patient will find it difficult to put their weight on their foot, and the ability to push off on the foot will become increasingly difficult. The patient will also not be able to rise onto their toes.

3) Diagnosis

Achilles ruptures are sometimes diagnosed by using the Thompson Technique. It was explained earlier in the book that your GP will ask you to lie face down and bend your knee; the doctor will then squeeze the calf muscles. If there is no plantar flexion, then it is likely that you have ruptured the tendon.

On some occasions the O'Brien test will be used. This technique involves having a needle inserted through the skin and into the tendon.

In some cases, it might be possible to tell that the Achilles has ruptured just by feeling along the back of the lower leg.

If it is thought likely that there is a rupture, the patient is likely to be sent for a scan. A Musculoskeletal ultrasonography will measure the thickness of a tendon and will show if there are any tears. An MRI scan will confirm if there is a rupture. MRI scans can also show Achilles tendinopathy and Achilles bursitis. X-rays are unlikely to be needed unless your doctor wants to rule out a fracture as tendons do not show in X- rays.

4) Achilles Tendon Rupture: Rehab and Treatment

Recent research has shown that surgery is not always necessary to repair the Achilles tendon and that casting the injured foot might be enough on its own. During surgery, the ruptured tendon will be stitched together, but researchers from Sweden discovered that this is not required to facilitate healing.

Katarina Nilsson Helander, MD, PhD at the Sahlgrenska Academy, University of Gothenburg, Sweden, headed a study to compare the results between patients who had surgery and those that didn't. 100 patients took part in the trial; half of them had surgery and early mobilisation, while the other half just had early mobilisation and wore a removable cast.

According to the study, there was no increased incidence of Achilles rupture in the patients who did not have their tendons surgically repaired.

The study author concluded that not every patient who ruptures an Achilles will need to have Achilles rupture surgery, but the patient would need to discuss the treatment options with their orthopaedic surgeon.

5) Achilles Tendon Rupture Recovery

Rehabilitating a ruptured tendon can be a long, painful process. Achilles tendon surgery recovery time can take anything from 4-12 months, and depending on how bad the damage is, it might not be possible to go back to the same level of activity as before the injury.

6) Insertional Tendonitis

The American Orthopaedic Foot and Ankle Society define Insertational Achilles tendonitis as a degeneration of the fibres of the Achilles as it inserts into the heel bone. This form of tendonitis can also be linked to Achilles bursitis and inflammation of the tendon sheaf.

As with other forms of tendonitis, the pain tends to come on slowly and the pain and swelling will be located at the insertion point of the Achilles. The pain will only usually become noticeable during activity to begin with, but if it goes untreated then the discomfort can continue to get worse until the pain becomes constant.

Causes

According to the American Orthopaedic Foot and Ankle Society, people aged forty or over, people with the skin condition psoriasis, Reiters syndrome and gout are among the people more prone to this type of tendonitis. It can also be associated with the use of steroids and some antibiotics.

Diagnosis

Insertational tendonitis is usually diagnosed by X-ray. However, an

MRI scan would give a better idea of just how damaged the tendon is and would also rule out other conditions such as bursitis.

Treatment

There are both surgical and non-surgical options for the treatment of this condition. Non-surgical options include NSAIDS such as Ibuprofen, heel lifts and stretching exercises.

The patient might also be advised to wear night splints and arch supports. It might also be suggested they attend physical therapy sessions.

Surgical

If non-surgical options fail then your consultant might suggest the possibility of surgery. Surgery involves removing the damaged part of the tendon, bone that might be causing irritation to the tendon, and if there is any inflammation in the bursa tissue, then this will also be removed.

Rehabilitation

Patients are likely to be in a splint for two weeks. After a six-eight week period, patients can then start work with a physiotherapist. It could take up to three months before it is possible to return to the sporting activities that a patient took part in before. If a tendon transfer was carried out during the operation, then recovery time can be significantly longer – lasting up to two years.

7) Achilles Bursitis

The causes of Achilles Bursitis are much the same as the causes behind tendonitis. Overuse and an increased amount of activity, which causes an additional strain on the Achilles that it isn't used to, can cause this condition.

About Achilles Bursitis

In Achilles Bursitis, the bursa sac within the heel becomes inflamed. Swelling is one of the main symptoms, and you are also likely to experience some pain in the ankle joint.

Symptoms

As with cases of tendonitis, the area is likely to feel tender to the touch, there will be swelling and you might notice that the area looks red. Pain is likely to become worse during increased activity.

Diagnosis

There is usually no need for any diagnostic tests to ascertain if a patient has bursitis. It is usually diagnosed through an examination where your doctor will look for areas of pain and tenderness. You'll be asked to flex your toes and bend them so your doctor can ascertain where the area of pain is.

Treatment

As with the early stages of Achilles tendinitis/tendinopathy, your doctor will advise rest and perhaps suggest that you use ice to help reduce the inflammation and swelling. Medications such as ibuprofen will also be prescribed. In addition, you might also be prescribed painkillers, if the discomfort is severe.

8) Achilles Tendinosis

When doctors use the term "Achilles tendinosis", they often mean that the tendon is showing signs of degeneration or there might be Achilles tears. However, some doctors also use this term to describe a tendon that just isn't healing very well.

Other medical professionals will call tendinosis "degenerative tendinopathy." While other medical professionals will use the terminology tendinitis or tendonitis; they are usually describing the same condition.

Diagnosis

Most patients with this condition will be in their mid-thirties and upwards. The tendon will show signs of swelling and the patient might find it difficult to walk. There won't usually be any need for scans as a doctor will determine if it is tendinosis just by examining the foot.

Treatment

Treatment options are unfortunately limited. As stated earlier in this book, Achilles tendons don't heal well and once injured it is all too easy to damage the tendon again.

If the symptoms are severe then a doctor might suggest wearing an Achilles walking boot or cast to rest the tendon. If the problem continues then surgical options will be discussed.

9) Achilles Lengthening

Achilles lengthening will usually be considered if a short tendon is contributing to your Achilles tendonitis and all other efforts to treat the condition have failed. It will also be considered if any of the following apply:

- If your Achilles is so tight that stretching isn't enough,

- If you have problems getting your heel to lower all of the way to the ground,

- The length of your Achilles is impeding how far you can flex your foot,

- If you have a foot drop that is caused by a short tendon, then your doctor might suggest looking at lengthening the tendon.

Achilles lengthening might also be offered as an option for patients suffering from tendonitis, flat feet or other types of foot deformities.

Achilles tendon lengthening is often carried out on younger people. Usually, more conservative methods of correcting the Achilles tendon will be made first. First of all, a doctor might suggest wearing a heel pad inside the shoe to see if this helps.

Later, and if there is no improvement from wearing the heel pad, then the patient will likely be sent to a physiotherapist where they will be prescribed various stretching exercises to try and increase tendon length.

If the problem with the Achilles tendon continues, then a surgeon or consultant might decide that it is time to start thinking about Achilles lengthening surgery.

Although none of the surgical procedures for Achilles lengthening sound pleasant, the surgery is usually straight forward, and when the foot comes out of the cast, bruising and signs of the surgery are usually minimal and not anything to be concerned about.

Although there will be some pain after this type of surgery, it is manageable, and painkillers such as paracetamol are likely to be prescribed.

The patient is likely to notice an ache in the back of the calf in the days and weeks after the surgery, and mobilisation after surgery might take a while. Provided all goes well, it shouldn't be too long after surgery that the patient can start getting back to normal, but care should be taken not to do anything that could cause sudden injury to the tendon as it will be pretty vulnerable following surgery.

There are several different surgical options when it comes to lengthening a tendon.

Percutaneous Method

A surgeon will make tiny cuts into the tendon. Over time, the cuts will heal and the tendon will lengthen. The tendon will then be stapled, or the surgeon might choose to use dissolving stitches. Sometimes the leg is then casted, but on other occasions a surgeon might choose just to bandage the affected area and advise the patients to wear an immobilisation boot while the tendon heals.

Gastroc Recession

In this type of surgery, the surgeon will make an incision into the gastrocnemius muscle in order to release it.

Z-Plasty Technique

This type of surgery will involve cutting the tendon at the halfway point and then making another incision up the middle of the tendon. Another slit will be made on the opposite side of the tendon and then the two sides of the tendon will be stitched together.

As with all surgery, there are some risks and these should be discussed with a surgeon beforehand. One concern is that once lengthened, the Achilles might just shorten or tighten up again over time. There is also a chance that the Achilles could be over lengthened, which might introduce a whole new set of problems. There is also the risk of infection or possible nerve damage. Achilles lengthening isn't something that should be entered into lightly, but it is something that is worth considering.

This type of surgery is usually carried out as a day case and a patient can typically expect to be in a plaster cast for six-eight weeks. Once the plaster has been removed, you'll be referred to a physiotherapist, who can help you regain the mobility you've lost during your time in cast and advice you on the stretches and strengthening exercises to do during your rehabilitation.

The therapist might also suggest some gentle exercises to build up the calf muscles that are likely to have atrophied while in cast. After a few week it is likely that you'll be advised to begin doing some more exercise such as walking; this will help maintain your fitness levels without causing too much stress on the tendon.

After the surgery, you will probably be left with a small scar at the back of the leg and after a while you might be able to feel a small piece of scar tissue, however, this should not impede your mobility in any way.

Although it might sound daunting, Achilles lengthening surgery is really quite common, and although there is some risk of complications, as mentioned before, the same can be said of all surgery.

If you are faced with the possibility of this type of surgery, then read all you can about it. The more you understand the procedure, the less frightening it will appear.

Results of this type of surgery and generally good and, provided you follow the doctors guidance, you should not face any real problems.

When it comes to surgical options, make sure that you know all there is to know about the procedure or the possible consequences of this type of surgery.

Chapter 3) After Your Injury

Once the patient feels ready to get back into exercise they'll need to take a few precautions to ensure that they don't overuse the tendon again or that they don't risk reinjuring the tendon in any other way.

Research recently published by the University of East Anglia shows that doing a moderate amount of exercise is good for overall tendon health. As the researchers make clear, too much exercise has often been associated as a contributor to tendon problems such as Achilles tendonitis. As Lead researcher Dr Eleanor Jones, from UEA's school of Biological Science, explained in a press release:

"The onset of tendon disease has always been associated with exercise, however this association has not been fully understood. We have shown that moderate exercise has a positive effect on tendons."

"In this study we talk about moderately high exercise and we would consider running to be moderately high. But it's important to remember that our research was carried out in the lab so to confirm this we would need to complete further clinical studies."

The research, which was published in *the Molecular Cell Research Journal*, showed that moderate activity decreased the level of metalloproteinase – an enzyme that has been associated with tendon disease.

The researchers have concluded that doing a limited amount of exercise can help and not hinder tendon health, however, more research is needed before the exact mechanics behind how activity is associated with tendon disease is fully understood.

When returning to exercise, it can be tempting to return to the kind of exercise that was being done before, however, the patient might find that they have more limitations after their injury and it might be necessary for their exercise routines to be very different from what they were before.

1) Get back into it slowly

Once a patient begins to exercise again they should only do a quarter or a half of what they would normally do. Don't push too hard too soon, or there is risk of causing further inflammation and swelling to an already vulnerable tendon.

Leave exercising for a couple days after your first session and see if there are any reactions. If there are, then avoid exercising until it is possible to exercise comfortably without any side effects.

Patients with Achilles pain also need to be aware that once they return to exercise, their muscles might be prone to spasm, which means they will tighten up more easily and also fatigue, making it difficult to exercise to the degree that they were before. Tight lower leg muscles can also change the way a person walks, causing the patient to pronate more. These are all things to be cautious of as they can add to the possibility of making the Achilles problem worse.

2) Warm Up and Cool Down

Ensure that the exercise routine incorporates a proper warm up and cool down session. Focus specifically on stretching the Achilles tendon, ankle and calf. It is also advisable to use an exercise band or a ProStretch band while you stretch to take some of the stress off the tendon.

It might also be useful to stop between sets when working on the lower legs and give the lower legs an additional stretch. For instance, complete one set of lunges then stop to stretch the calves, shins and Achilles before continuing with the second set. This will help to avoid the muscles tightening up too much during a workout.

Cooling down is also vital after exercise. Not only does a cool down session help prevent the blood from pooling and lowers heart rate and pulse rate, it helps reduce the tightness and tension accumulated during the exercise sessions.

Finish your fitness routine by reducing the pace gradually and march on the spot until you feel your heart rate come down to normal. When your heart rate has slowed sufficiently, stretch the muscles, concentrating on the lower body area, as well as any of the other areas worked during exercise.

3) Wear proper sports shoes

Wearing proper sports shoes is essential for helping to avoid re-injury, and for preventing injury in the first place. Improper footwear that does not offer enough support to the foot during exercise is one of the most common causes of Achilles tendonitis. Ideally, you should buy a pair of sports shoes that give your ankles support and that offer additional arch support.

Buy shoes that are designed for your type of sports. Running, tennis etc., all require a different level of support as they all put different stresses on the feet.

If pronation is a problem then get advice from a sports store about choosing a pair of trainers that are designed to help control the inward roll of your foot as you run or walk.

If the support offered by the trainers isn't enough and the foot still rolls inward when taking part in activity, then you are likely to benefit from orthotics or inserts.

4) Listen to your Body

After recovering from Achilles injury it is important to take special care to not reinjure the tendon or to do anything that could put stress or strain on the Achilles as once the tendon has been injured, it is far easier to injure it again. Also, if the health of the tendon isn't good, it can take much longer to heal should it become injured again.

Once you are back into your old exercise routine, you should be mindful of any pain or of the previous symptoms of the tendonitis. If some of the old symptoms return- no matter how minor - the patient should stop exercising and rest.

If it proves difficult to get back into your previous exercise routine without causing pain, then it is best to consult a sports therapist who can give advice on the kind of exercises to do and the amount of repetitions. This will differ from person to person.

5) Learn your trigger points

Most people will have some idea of the factors that contribute to their Achilles problems. If the cause is due to repetitive actions then you'll need to reduce the amount of repetitions or introduce stretching to the regular routine to break up the repetitious nature.

If using heavy weights has contributed to the condition, then you'll need to look at changing your routine and lifting lighter weights to avoid putting too much strain on an already over-worked Achilles.

If you know there is going to be a lot of repetitive activity that can't be avoided, then try using kinesiology tape to strap the ankle and support the Achilles tendon.

Kinesiology tape is used by some of the world's top athletes and was worn by many sports stars at London 2012 and at Wimbledon. The tape gives additional support to joints and tendons, doesn't mark the skin in the same way that some sports' tapes do, and will stay on for several days even if it gets wet.

Before using kinesiology tape, it is vital that you learn how to strap the Achilles properly, as a poorly strapped ankle or Achilles will put additional stress on the foot. A sports therapist will be able to show you how to strap the foot to help avoid injury and to reduce pronation as you exercise. This will reduce the level of stress on the Achilles as well as the ankle..

6) Change your Routine

Doing the same routine day in day out is almost guaranteed to cause excessive stress to the tendons. When exercising it is best to avoid working the same body part every day so it is best to focus on lower body exercises one day and upper body exercises the next day to avoid overuse. There should also be at least a couple of stretch days every week to ensure that the muscles do not get too tight. Depending on how bad the tendonitis is, it might also be advisable to look at taking up an entirely different sport, especially if the activity you would normally partake in involves a lot of strenuous or repetitive exercise.

7) Sports Taping

If you know there is going to be a lot of repetitive activity that can't be avoided, then try using kinesiology tape to strap the ankle and support the Achilles tendon.

Kinesiology tape is used by some of the world's top athletes and was worn by many sports stars at London 2012 and at Wimbledon. The tape gives additional support to joints and tendons, doesn't mark the skin in the same way that some sports' tapes do, and will stay on for several days even if it gets wet.

Another advantage of this type of tape is that it has been designed to support tendons and will help take the stress off them while they slowly start to heal. Using the tape can also help relieve some of the pain from Achilles tendon by giving the tendon the addition support it needs while it heals.

This type of sports tape is also affordable so it should be within most people's price range if they want a cost effective way to try and keep some of their tendon problems at bay.

Kinesiology tape can also be bought ready cut, making the task of applying it – and of making sure it is cut correctly – just a little bit easier, however, the manufacturers of such products advise that it is still better to get the tape professionally applied. In addition, the ready-cut tapes are only designed for one off usage, so if you need to strap your foot up regularly so that you can take part in sports, then you might find it expensive. In that case, buying the tape is a better option.

Before using kinesiology tape, it is vital that you learn how to strap the Achilles properly, as a poorly strapped ankle or Achilles will put additional stress on the foot. A sports therapist will be able to show you how to strap the foot to help avoid injury and to reduce pronation as you exercise. This will reduce the level of stress on the Achilles as well as the ankle or you can buy books on how to strap a foot to help reduce wear and tear, however, you really need to be confident with what you are doing before attempting to strap your own feet.

8) Sports Massage

Often, just stretching the tendons and muscles isn't enough and the power of massage is often underestimated. In order to really get into the muscles and reduce the tension that can contribute to Achilles problems, a sports massage will help get rid of deep seated tension.

Many athletes depend on massage therapy to help keep their muscles limber and the amateur athlete can benefit from it too. A good massage will help loosen up muscles after an intense gym session and can help keep aches and pains at bay. It can also reduce tightness to help ensure that your muscles don't get so tight that they go into spasm, which is common with over-worked, over used muscles.

Reducing the tension in the muscles plays a vital part in the reduction of stress on the tendons, thus people with Achilles tendonitis will find a regular massage valuable to them.

There are several types of massage that can be used. The ideal type of massage will be one that prepares the muscles properly for intense activity or a type of massage that will work to elongate the muscles and reduce tension following an exercise session. You'll find a chapter on various massage techniques later on in this book.

Chapter 4) Exercises

When doing stretches for the Achilles tendon it is also important to stretch other muscles and tendons. Often, tight calves can contribute to Achilles tendonitis, and weak calves can cause the condition tendonitis as well.

As detailed earlier on in the book, pronation will also place an additional strain on the Achilles because of the constant pull on the muscles and tendons; weak arches or flat feet will also play a role in the development of Achilles tendonitis or tendinopathy.

Detailed in this chapter is a set of exercises which are designed especially to loosen and strengthen the calves, shins and Achilles tendon. There are also some additional exercises to strengthen the arches, which might help to reduce pronation, thus reducing the strain on the Achilles tendon. However, before exercising, it is wise to get some advice from your GP or a sports therapist as they will be able to advise you on which exercises are best suited to you.

Before beginning the stretches it is advisable to gently warm up first. This could be anything from some gentle marching on the spot or a short walk, anything that will get the blood flowing and make the tendons and muscles easier to stretch.

The stretches described concentrate on the lower leg muscles, however, if you are prone to tendonitis then you'll find a workout that stretches and isolates each muscle and tendon helpful in reducing tension throughout the body. There are plenty of stretch DVDs available that will provide a 20-30 minute routine and target the major muscles; stretch cards are also available so you can choose the few from the deck that you need to do the most. A stretch routine should be part of your weekly workout to help reduce tightness and tension that accumulates in muscles when you exercise.

Some of stretches can be carried out using the Medi-Dyne Pro-Stretch. This product is ideal for making sure that your foot stays properly aligned during the exercise and allows a deeper stretch to be achieved. The Pro-Stretch will also help to strengthen the ankles, which might be helpful in cases of ankle instability.

The Medi-Dyne Pro-Stretch is available from Amazon and from online stores in the UK and US.

If you feel any pain during these exercises then you should stop the move straight away. If in doubt, consult an expert before beginning any new strength and stretching exercises following an injury.

1) Eccentric Calf Exercises

Several studies have shown eccentric calf training to be effective in helping people cope with some of the symptoms of Achilles tendinopathy, and it will also help to reduce pain and increase mobility. There were some concerns that this type of training could affect the micro circulation to the Achilles, however, another study seems to have allayed fears over this.

An illustration of how to carry out these types of exercises has been made available by the NHS in Sheffield. http://www.sheffield.nhs.uk/podiatry/resources/pilcalfstreng thening.pdf

These exercises should not be attempted without first getting advice to ensure that these exercises are safe for you to do.

2) Calf and Achilles stretch

Face the wall and stand with your toes against the wall. Step back with your right foot so that your heel is on the ground. Next, lean forward using your arms to press into the wall and feel the stretch all the way down to the back of the leg. The stretch should be held for up to 30 seconds and then repeated on the left side.

Each stretch should be completed three times.

3) Alternative Calf Stretch

If you didn't feel much of a stretch in the last exercise, this could be due to excessive tightness in the calves or Achilles. If this is the case, then push your weight onto the outer edges of your foot. This should give a more powerful stretch, but you need to take care with this in case it is too much for an already vulnerable tendon. The stretch should only be held for a short while; long enough to feel the effects but not so long that it causes pain.

4) Another Calf Stretch

Using a stair or step to support you, place your toes on the edge of the step so that your heel is hanging off of the step and tilt your foot backwards off the step so just the front part of your foot remains on. This will give a much deeper stretch, but should be approached with caution if you are still recovering from injury.

By bending the back leg, it is possible to get a stretch in the muscles lower down, so you'll be able to target a tight Achilles tendon this way, too, but be careful not to put undue pressure on the Achilles.

5) Soleus Stretch

The Soleus muscle runs from below the knee and into the heel. The Soleus is using in everyday actions such as walking and standing. It is not often that this muscle gets much of a stretch, but as it is so closely situated to the calf, it is important to focus on this area, too.

Directions:

Place one foot so that it is flat against the wall. The other foot should be behind you and bent at the knee. Hold this stretch for up to thirty seconds and then repeat the move on the other side. This exercise should be repeated three times on each leg, however, if you find this stretch makes the back of your knee sore, reduce the amount of times you do this exercise.

6) Tibia Stretch

The Tibia anterior muscle is at the front of the lower leg and is essential for the dorsiflexion of your foot as you walk. It also helps to invert the foot. As you have stretched the muscles of the back of the leg, it is important to also focus on the muscles at the front so that you don't create an imbalance between the muscles, which could lead to a tightening in the shin and make it difficult to lift your foot.

When your foot is held in a plantar flexion or pointed position, this stretches the muscle down the front of the leg. To stretch this muscle you can either sit with your legs straight out in front of you either on the bed or the floor. Point your toes until they touch the floor. You should feel this move in the front of your leg. Repeat three times, but do fewer repetitions if it is making your muscles ache.

7) Alternative Version

Stand up with your legs slightly apart, one slightly in front of the other. Step backward on your right leg and press your toes into the ground. You should feel a stretch running up through your shin muscle. The stretch should be held for 30 seconds, less if you feel pain or discomfort.

The above exercise is also useful if you suffer from tight shins or shin splits and can help you lift your foot better when you walk.

8) Calf Raises

A weakness in the lower calf muscles is often associated with Achilles problems. In this next series of exercises, we'll look at exercises to help improve the strength in the calf area. Cycling and stepping are also good ways of building calf muscles, however, neither of these should be attempted if you are still struggling through an injury of any sort.

If your leg muscles have atrophied following an injury, then these moves can help to gently build up bulk. You might also like to take protein powder or amino acids to help make the exercises more effective.

9) Calf Raise

Stand with your feet together and rise onto your toes. Contract the muscles right at the top and when you come back down, contract the muscles again. Repeat this exercise at least five times and then work up to thirty.

10) Alternatives

If your aim is to improve the strength on the inside of your calves, then point your toes inward when you rise onto your toes. If you want to build muscle on the outside of the calves, then point your toes outward.

11) Single Leg Calf Raise

As well as building strength in the calf, this move helps to improve balance and ankle strength. If you are recovering from an injury, then you need to ensure that this move does not cause you pain, so begin with low repetitions and stretch out **the calves and shins in between each set to make sure that your muscles don't get too tight.**

60

Directions:

Hook your left leg around your right calf and rise up onto your toes. Hold the move until you feel a contraction at the peak of the exercise, and then lower your foot to the ground. As you lower, squeeze the muscle again to work the muscle a little bit harder.

Repeat this move at least five times and then change to the left side. Remember to stretch your calves and shins after completing this exercise.

12) Squat Variation

This move was adapted after an Achilles injury. The aim with this move was to build up calf muscle, but to avoid putting too much strain onto the Achilles tendon. Stand against the bed so that your lower legs are against the bed. Lower down to just above the bed and then raise back up, squeezing the buttock muscles as you do.

You should feel this exercise in the calves; this is one of the most effective ways of isolating them and working the muscles harder. Only do a few repetitions of these as they are hard on the muscles and the aim is to avoid overworking the Achilles.

13) Seated Calf Raise

Sit up straight on a sturdy chair, a sofa, or a bed. Place your hands on the knees to provide some gentle resistance. Next lift your heels up until your feet are on tip toes and hold the move until you feel the contraction in your calf. Repeat at least 10 times.

14) Calf Raise with Ball

Hold a tennis ball in between your ankles. Rise up onto your feet as you would with the calf raise. Hold the move until you feel a contraction in your calves then lower back down. Using a tennis ball allows proper alignment of the feet and can help to prevent pronation.

Repeat the move at least 10 times.

15) Seated Toe Tap

The shin area isn't a part of the body that gets exercised very often. This simple exercise will provide a simple way of working the shins. Remember to stretch the shins out afterwards.

Directions:

Sit up straight on a chair or a bed. Your feet should be flat on the ground. Flex the feet towards you so you feel a contraction in the shins. Tap the toe to the floor and then repeat the exercise at least ten times.

16) Arch Exercises

If your feet pronate or you have flat feet or weak arches then this will leave you vulnerable to Achilles problems. It will also increase the chances of developing Plantar Fasciitis – a painful inflammation of the plantar tendon that runs along the bottom of your foot and into your toe. It will also leave you vulnerable to shin splints, which is another common sports injury.

If you do have problems with your arches, then you'll need to speak to a sports therapist or podiatrist who can best advise you on some support to wear. If you want to try and strengthen your arches, then here are some simple exercises.

17) Towel Scrunch

Put a towel in front of you and use your toes to scrunch up the towel bit by bit, squeezing the arches as you do. Repeat this exercise as many times as is comfortable. This exercise is also suitable for people prone to ankle sprains.

18) Arch Scrunch

This is another exercise designed to strengthen your arches.

Directions:

Sit up straight with your feet flat on the floor and scrunch your arch, making it appear higher. Hold for a few seconds and then release.

A product called the Elgin Archxerciser is also available. This will enable you do the same move, but the exercise is more effective than using a towel. These products have a limited availability in the UK, but they can be ordered from sports stores in the US.

19) Tennis Ball Roll

This exercise will help to provide relief for anyone with painful Plantar Fasciitis. It will also point and flex your feet, gently stretching your calves and shins.

Directions:

Place a tennis ball or rolling pin underneath your foot and roll your foot along the ball all of the way forward until your toe reaches a point, then roll it all of the way back until your foot flexes. Repeat this exercise as often as you like.

This exercise is also good for releasing tension in the lower leg area and in the arches. Make the movements slow so that you can enjoy the feel of the ball massaging the sole of your foot.

20) Alphabets

Alphabets are a simple, fun exercise that builds the arches as well as strengthening the ankles and improving balance. As well as being suitable for people with Achilles injuries, this is also good for people with plantar fasciitis or with ankles that have been weakened from sprains and strains.

Directions

Sit on the edge of the bed. Sit far back enough so that your feet are off the floor. Draw the alphabet with your foot, one letter at a time, ensuring that you take your ankle through the complete range of motion to get the most out of the exercise.

Repeat as many times as is comfortable.

21) Arch Exercise

This exercise will help strengthen the arch of the foot and also helps after ankle injury. This exercise might also reduce pronation if practiced often enough.

Sit in the same position as you did for the alphabet. Begin with your feet pointing forwards. Turn your feet inwards until your toes meet each other and then return back to their original position.

22) Standing Arch Exercises

Stand with your feet close together then push your weight onto the outsides of your feet. Repeat this exercise up to 30 times.

Another way of helping to reduce pronation is sitting with your feet out in front of you and resting them on the outer edges of your feet. You can stay in this position for as long as you find comfortable, but be careful not to hold it for too long or you risk the lower leg muscles tightening up and going into spasm.

23) Ankle Exercises

People with Achilles pain can also be prone to pain in their ankles. It is also possible that an Achilles injury will begin to reduce the mobility in the ankle. These exercises will help to keep the ankles mobile.

Ashtanga yoga provides a good way of stretching and strengthening the ankles and lower leg muscles. You could also try using a rowing machine to encourage the development of the calf and shin muscles.

24) Ankle Circles

Lie back on a bed with your feet pointing straight up towards the ceiling. Circle your ankles clockwise five times and then repeat anti-clockwise. This exercise will also help to loosen the lower leg muscles.

25) Flexi Band Exercises

Hook a flexi band around the arches of your feet. Point your feet against the band until your feet are pointed as far as they can comfortably go. Next, flex your feet back towards you to complete the move. Repeat this exercise as often as is comfortable.

26) Toe Exercises

Maintaining strength and flexibility in your toes can help your balance and strengthen your push off as you walk. This can give you more stability and will aid your mobility. It will also help to build the arches and increase the overall strength of the muscles in your toes.

Sit on a chair or the edge of a bed. Take a pen and try and pick it up with your toes. Repeat this exercise ten times. You can also do this exercise with marbles, bits of paper or bean bags.

27) Toe Stretches

Take your toes in your hand and use your fingers to gently stretch your toes out. This is an ideal exercise for people if they have toes that are starting to "claw" as it will help to stretch out the tendons. If done regularly, it should help keep the tendons in your toes from tightening up any further. This exercise is also good for practicing in water.

28) Toe Pulls

Hook an elastic band around your big toes then pull them away from each other. Repeat at least five times.

29) Balance Exercises

If you've had a lower leg injury then you might have noticed that your balance becomes affected. This could be because you have lost some muscle in the injured leg. You can help to compensate for this by practicing balancing on the weaker leg for as long as you can or you could try some of the balance poses that you'll find in yoga.

A balance board is also a good way of building ankle strength and learning to get your balance back. While practicing on this, you also have the option of pushing your weight onto the outside of your feet to try and help reduce pronation.

30) Ankle and Hip Stretch

A tight hip flexor can make you more likely to walk with your foot averted. As well as putting a strain on the hip, this will also put an additional stress on the ankle. This stretch helps to loosen up both the ankle and hip.

Directions: Sit up straight on a sturdy chair or on a bed. Rest your left ankle gently on your right knee. Be careful not to put too much stress on the knee joint when you do this. Push lightly with the inside of your foot until you feel a stretch in the ankle and hip. Hold for up to 30 seconds or for as long as is comfortable. Repeat on the other side.

The exercises in this chapter should not just be practiced when you are recovering from injury. Although these stretches can help to loosen muscles and stretch tendons, they are not just for use when undergoing Achilles tendon treatment or Achilles tendon rehab and they can help prevent injury.

Chapter 5) Yoga Therapy

Yoga therapy was touched upon briefly in an earlier chapter. However, the subject of yoga therapy is worth delving into a little deeper as it can be extremely beneficial to people with Achilles tendon problems, provided it is practiced safely and carefully. Yoga should not be practiced while the tendon is still painful as stretching is likely to make the pain worse.

Many athletes - Andy Murray among them – practice yoga to improve their strength and flexibility, and they no doubt benefit from the mental benefits of yoga, too.

It would be advisable to consult a sports therapist or a yoga therapist first to ensure that you get the best out of the moves and that you don't risk any damage to your tendon.

If you are used to working your muscles hard then yoga will provide a much gentler alternative as your Achilles begins to heal. It will help to stretch the tendons as well as help reduce tension throughout the body. Yoga is also great for improving the alignment of the muscles and improving posture, which will help you to stand better and move better, thus reducing the strain on the Achilles.

Yoga can also be used as a workout on its own if you practice the Ashtanga version, which burns fat as well as helping to tone muscles and stretch muscles and tendons. Yoga can be more effective at stretching the tendons as it gives a more prolonged, concentrated stretch. Care should be taken not to over stretch the tendons and before starting to practice yoga you'll need to consult your GP to get some advice on if yoga is right for your personal circumstances.

Yoga also provides a more intense stretch than the usual stretches that are performed before and after exercise. It is also believed that yoga can help to eliminate toxins, improve circulation, and lift general well-being. Certainly, regular practice will make the muscles and tendons more flexible and help avoid some of the postural or alignment problems that are known to contribute to Achilles tendonitis.

If you haven't stretched for a while then you might also find that when you first start to practice yoga, your muscles tighten up. This is normal as the tendons will bunch up to protect themselves from further injury, however, consistency is the key and the more you practice, the easier it will become.

If you have biomechanical problems such as pronation, yoga can also be used to help reduce the inward roll of your foot by pushing your weight onto the outsides of your feet as you practice the moves. It can also be used to strengthen the arches, which will also help to reduce the stress on the Achilles.

1) Ashtanga Yoga

People with very tight muscles won't find stretching enough on its own; however, Ashtanga yoga can provide a more intense stretch as well as improving your posture and helping to maintain your fitness level. If Ashtanga Yoga isn't for you, then there is always the option of trying the more relaxed Hatha Yoga. Again, stretching your muscles by practicing this type of yoga will provide a much more intense stretch than the stretching people would normally do after exercising. The same muscles and tendons are often repeatedly stretched out during different postures, but be careful that this doesn't cause soreness or pain in the injured tendon.

Poses such as the triangle, warrior, seated forward bend and single leg stretch will all help to increase flexibility in the lower legs and Sun Salutations - a series of yoga moves that can be used as a warm up - will help stretch out the entire body. Downward dog will give the calves, ankles and Achilles a deep stretch. If you push your weight onto the outside of the feet while in this pose it can help strengthen the ankles, reducing stress on the tendon.

If you are new to Ashtanga yoga, then learn all you can about it, and learn how to use it to its best benefits. When starting out, take your time, and don't be too surprised if yoga takes more out of you than you thought possible.

Although Ashtanga yoga can be energy boosting, if it is practiced wrongly, then it can be very draining as well. Ashtanga yoga will make you sweat so it will also help to draw out toxins from your body, too.

You need to be careful not to make your Achilles sore by stretching too deeply and if you have been recently injured and your tendon still hurts, then don't do Ashtanga yoga as it will be too much.

Remember to pace yourself when taking part in your yoga practice and stop at the first point of pain. Make sure that you listen to your body, and while you should expect this type of yoga to be a challenge, don't push yourself too hard or you will increase your risk of injury all over again.

Moves can typically be held for 15-30 seconds, but care should be taken not to cause yourself any pain and the moves should only be held for as long as comfortable. To practice yoga comfortably, there are a few things you should do:

1. Wear loose clothing, making sure that the temperature is not too cold or too cold.

2. Find a time when you know you won't be disturbed so you can take your time to relax into the poses and get the most out of them.

3. Only stretch as far as you can go and don't stretch until the point of soreness.

4. Keep plenty of water handy.

5. Make sure you have a towel and a non-slip yoga mat.

6. Most people practice yoga barefoot, however, there are yoga socks and yoga shoes now available.

2) Cobbler Pose

Sit erect with your legs out straight then bend your knees outwards so that your soles are together and exhale as you move forward into the posture. Put some light pressure on the outside of your feet to help intensify the stretch. Inhale to come out of the pose. Cobbler pose will help relax the ankles and feet, stretch out tight and tense back muscles, and relax the hip and groin area.

If you can't get your knees all of the way down to the floor, then don't strain. Instead use a folded towel to rest your knees on. As your flexibility develops, the posture will become easier.

After completing Cobbler pose, you can release your legs so they are extended in front of you and then move into forward bend or single leg stretch, if you wish.

Precautions: Care should be taken if you have shoulder or hip problems.

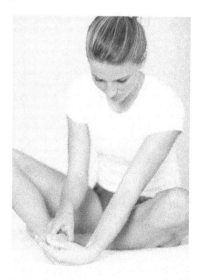

3) Chair Pose

Chair pose will help to stretch a tight Achilles tendon as well as develop strength in the lower leg muscles. It will also improve balance and increase strength in the thigh muscles.

Take a deep breath, raise your hands above your head and then bend at the knees as you slowly lower yourself as if you were going to sit down. This move can be held for up to 30 seconds, but beginners can try holding the move for 8-10 seconds. Avoid this move if you have hip or knee problems.

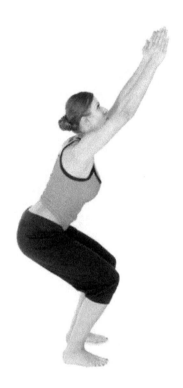

4) Big Toe Pose

Stand up straight with your feet slightly apart. Your feet should be far enough apart to provide a gentle stretch, but not so far apart that you lose your stability or risk stretching too far. Take a breath in and gently lower yourself forward and hold each of your big toes with your fingers. Once in this position, see if you can straighten your arms/elbows; take an inhale before you do.

If you are unable to stretch all of the way down then bend forward until your hands reaching your hamstrings. This will provide a moderate stretch and won't be so challenging on the hamstrings or the back of the legs.

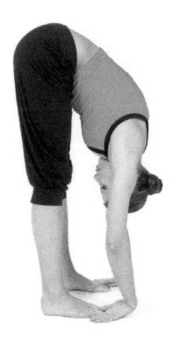

5) Thunder Pose

This pose helps to strengthen the arches and stretch the ankles. Caution should be taken with this pose if you suffer from knee pain. If your ankle hurts when you attempt this posture then come out of the move.

Kneel on the floor with your knees together and the feet slightly apart. The soles of your feet should point upwards to the ceiling as you sit back on your buttocks.

Precautions:

This posture can cause pain in the knees and ankles if not practiced properly. If you have knee or ankle problems, take advice before practicing this move.

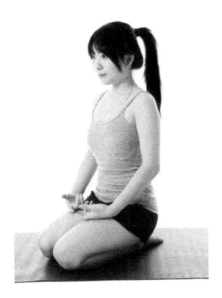

6) Warrior Pose

As you breathe out, step your feet until they are 3-4 feet apart. Lift your arms out to the sides. Your left foot should be turned in to a 45 degree angle and your right foot should be positioned at a 90 degree angle. Twist your torso to face your right foot and then bend your right knee forward. Take care to ensure that your knee does not reach past your foot to avoid putting excessive strain on your knee joints. Hold the pose for up to 30 seconds and inhale as you come up.

The pose can then be repeated to the other side.

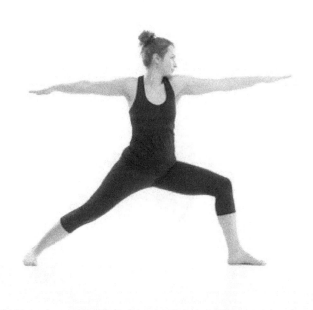

7) Triangle

With an exhale, step your feet until they are 3-4 feet apart. Turn your left foot to a 45 degree angle and your right foot out to a 90 degree angle. As you breathe in slide your right arm down to your right leg until your hand reaches your ankle while gently extending your left arm at an angle. Turn your head to look up at the left hand and hold the pose for up to 30 seconds. If you have neck problems, don't look up at your hand; instead stare down at your right foot. Take an inhale to come back up and then repeat the move on the other side.

Precautions: People with back problems should avoid this move or take care when they practice. People will neck problems should also be careful not to put a strain on their neck muscles. It should also be avoided by people who suffer with headaches or migraines.

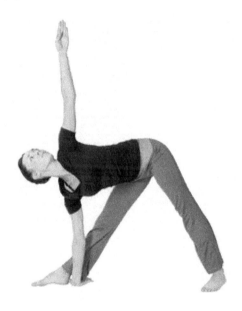

8) Seated Forward Bend

As well as stretching the back of the legs, this yoga move will also help to release tight back muscles and will help calm the mind after a long day.

Directions:

Sit up straight with both legs straight out in front of you. Inhale as you raise both arms until they are straight above your head, then on the exhale lean forward and take hold of the soles of your feet. If you don't have enough flexibility to do this then use a yoga belt or an exercise band. Deepen the stretch by inhaling again and exhaling to relax further into the pose. Hold the move for up to thirty seconds. Inhale to come up.

Precautions: This move should not be attempted if you have back, leg or shoulder problems.

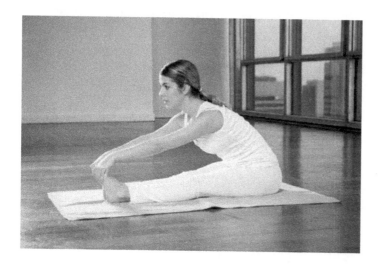

9) Downward Dog

Downward Dog can be used on its own or as part of the Sun Salutation set of postures. The Downward Dog posture will stretch the Achilles and calves, your shoulders and your chest, and will also help to calm your mind.

This posture also provides an ideal opportunity to push the weight gently to the outside of your feet; if you suffer from pronation then you will benefit greatly from this powerful but simple stretch.

You can get into this posture by kneeling, then reaching your hands forward, breathe out and gradually lift your knees. Press your hands firmly into the ground and continue to straighten your hands and knees until you reach the inverted V position.

To come out of this posture, gently lower your knees back to the floor.

Precautions: Care should be taken not to lock the knees or the elbows while in this posture. Avoid this move if you have wrist, shoulder, arm, back or hip problems.

If you suffer from high blood pressure or are prone to headaches or migraines then you should take medical advice before practicing downward dog or any of the inverted postures.

These are just a limited amount of yoga postures that can help stretch the Achilles tendon. By watching DVDs, buying books or attending yoga classes, you can see just how many of the poses could be used to stretch the tendon.

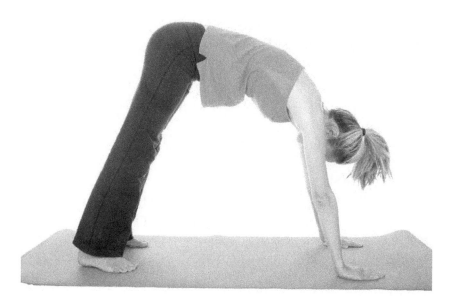

Chapter 6) Sports Massage

Often, just stretching the tendons and muscles isn't enough, especially when training regularly and when excessive loads are put on the tendon. In order to really get into the muscles and reduce the tension that can contribute to Achilles problems, a sports massage is necessary.

Massage is something you could try yourself by following the many massage techniques described in books and DVDs and using a basic sports massage therapy lotion. however, it is best to get a qualified sports therapist to do this as this type of massage is not nearly as effective as getting a trained therapist to work on your muscles.

A therapist will also be able to detect any other areas of tightness that might contribute to your Achilles problem.

A sports therapist can concentrate mainly on the calf and ankle area to help stop the muscles tightening up, reduce tension, and to help the limbs move more freely.

Here is an introduction to the types of massage that might be of benefit for those struggling with a sports injury.

Massage has the following benefits:

- It can boost healing by increasing circulation

- It can help reduce the spasms from tight muscles

- It can relax the muscles

- It will improve the range of motion in the joints, allowing you to move easier

- It will stretch out tight muscles

- It will help ease muscles that are sore from being overused.

A heated massager can help reduce spasms in muscles that have a tendency to tighten up easily. Tight muscles in the lower leg can make a person walk more plantar flexed or on their tip toes, thus causing stress to the Achilles. This type of walking will also cause excessive stress to the plantar tendon.

Using a heated massager for just a few minutes before and after exercising can help reduce this tightness and it can also be used on days when you feel that your muscles are tighter than others, and your range of motion feels more limited.

Heated massagers should not be used by people with diabetes, poor circulation, neurological conditions, or anyone who has reduced feeling in their feet or legs.

1) Kneading Massage

A kneading massage is often used to prepare the muscles ahead of taking part in sports events or other forms of exercise. This kind of massage helps to warm up muscles, boost circulation, and prepares the muscles for the challenges ahead.

2) Deep Tissue Massage

If the aim is to loosen tight muscles, eliminate toxins and to boost circulation, then deep tissue massage is a good choice. It can be used as an all over massage technique, however, a therapist can also focus on just the injured area or the surrounding area, if the injury is too tender to touch.

3) Swedish Massage

Swedish Massage is used to help relax the muscles. If your sports involves a lot of repetitive actions or requires you to repeatedly bear heavy loads, then this type of massage might be the most beneficial.

4) Heated Massage

This type of massage is also useful to reducing lactic acid in the body and enables the body to cope better with fatigue. Swedish massage will also help to limit stiffness and is useful after strenuous bouts of exercise.

5) Shiatsu Massage

As well as the relaxing effect this kind of massage has, it is also thought to promote a feeling of well-being. It is believed that shiatsu massage will help the flow of the body's energy. Shiatsu massage is carried out while the patient is fully clothed and the technique involves the use of stretches, finger pressure and palm pressure.

6) Manual Lymphatic Drainage Massage

This type of massage is useful if there is a lot of swelling following your Achilles injury. The massage will encourage the swelling around the Achilles to reduce and will also reduce swelling around the ankle area.

7) Cross Friction Massage

Some people recommend an intensive course of cross friction massage to help heal the discomfort of Achilles tendonitis. However, this type of massage can cause pain for some people, especially if the tendon is already feeling tender to the touch.

As this type of massage is extremely intense it is not recommended while the pain is at its worst and cross friction massage should not be carried out every day.

8) Effleurage Massage

Effleurage Massage involves using gentle strokes against the skin and might be suitable for people who have suffered from a recent injury. It is often used as a technique to warm up the muscles before other massage techniques are applied, but this type of gentle massage can be used on its own and it can be used against small areas of the body.

9) Petrissage

This is a form of kneading massage. It works deep into the muscles so it might be a little too harsh for people with recent injuries. However, it is an effective way of ridding tension from the body and can be used on the lower legs.

Chapter 7) Vitamins and Minerals

When it comes to treating tendon problems, some people prefer the more natural approach and start to look towards vitamins, minerals and supplements in a bid to heal the pain and discomfort caused by Achilles injuries. However, research on just how effective supplements might be is mixed, and some people get better results than others.

Most vitamins and supplements are affordably priced, so it can be worth considering taking a supplement and seeing if it does indeed have a positive effect on the symptoms of tendonitis.

There have been many studies carried out into minerals and how they might help the healing process in tendonitis, however, many of these studies are very limited and are often limited to animal models.

Anyone considering taking supplements should first talk to their GP or consultant and ensure that the supplements they intend to take will not interact with any other medication that might have been prescribed.

1) Magnesium and tendonitis

Dr, Carolyn Dean, MD, ND, is the author of "The Magnesium Miracle" and she believes that a lack of magnesium can contribute to a range of illnesses and conditions.

Dr. Dean believes that a lack of the mineral magnesium plays a significant role in the development of tendonitis and suggests that a lack of magnesium will contribute to tendonitis before a patient becomes aware of it. Dr Dean also believes that a lack of magnesium plays a part in both new cases of newly established

84

tendonitis as well as in chronic, on-going cases of tendonitis.

Dr. Dean explains that when a person carries out repetitive actions such as such as baseball, the body uses up large quantities of magnesium, which often aren't replaced by the daily diet.

While some people disagree with this theory, it should be noted that magnesium does help tight muscles to relax. If a patient has tight, tense muscles, this can then put an additional strain on the tendons and contribute to the pain and inflammation.

It is recommended that patients do not take more than 900mg of magnesium a day. Some experts recommend that patients who take calcium as well as magnesium can experience depleted levels of magnesium so they suggest taking calcium and magnesium at a ratio of 2:1. Supplements are available. However, some experts argue that extra calcium isn't needed and there have been several health alerts relating to calcium supplementation recently and it is best to get expert advice before taking supplements.

Recommended Daily Intake:

19-30 years 360mg for women and 410mg for men

31-50 years 320mg for women and 420mg for men

51 and over 320mg for women and 420mg for men

Food Sources:

Nuts, seeds, beans, yogurt, spinach, rice, salmon, milk and broccoli.

Precautions:

Too much magnesium can cause stomach cramps, nausea and digestive upsets.

People taking diuretics, antibiotics or Proton pump inhibitors should take medical advice before supplementing with magnesium.

2) Vitamin C

Vitamin C is important to the health of collagen, which makes it vital to the health of tendons. A study carried out in 2009 by the Department of Histology and Embryology, Faculty of Medicine in Gaza University, Turkey showed that vitamin C could increase the acceleration of healing following a rupture of the Achilles tendon. The study was carried out on rats; the rodents were given vitamin C in high doses once every two days. Of the 42 rodents used in the study, half of them were given 150mgs of vitamin C every two days. The group given the vitamin C showed an improvement after three days. After 21 days, collagen levels were increased and damaged tissue was quicker to repair.

The researchers concluded that the vitamin C had accelerated healing and there was an increased collagen synthesis in the rat models. Further studies are to be carried out into the role vitamin C can play in the healing of Achilles tendon problems.

Sources:

Vitamin C is found in fruits, vegetables and juices. If taking supplements, Vitamin C should be limited to once a day.

Precautions:

Vitamin C is generally safe to take. However, high doses could affect iron, B12 and copper levels.

People taking statins or undergoing cancer treatment should take advice before taking vitamin C.

Recommended Daily Doses:

65mg for females aged 13-18

75mg for females aged 19 and over

75mg for males aged 13-18

90mg for males aged 19 and over

3) Vitamin E

The anti-oxidant vitamin E is known to have anti-inflammatory effects and may help reduce pain and swelling. However, vitamin e should not be taken by patients on blood thinning drugs and diabetics need to take care as it can cause lower blood sugar levels. If you have prescription medication, consult your doctor before taking vitamin E.

Sources:

Vitamin E is found in vegetables oils, margarine, nuts, seeds and green vegetables. Recommended daily amounts vary between 4mg and 19mg a day, depending on age.

Precautions:

High doses of vitamin E are not recommended for diabetics. Patients with heart conditions should also be careful when taking vitamin E. Cancer patients, patients on anticoagulant or anti-platelet medications and statins should take medical advice before supplementing with vitamin E.

4) Vitamin B6

A lack of vitamin B6 can influence the inflammatory processes. If you decide to take to take B vitamins, it is best to take them as part of a B complex as taking one vitamin on its own may deplete other B vitamins.

Sources:

B6 is found in grains, cereals, bread, pulses, fish, turkey and oats.

Doses:

The recommended daily amount for B6 starts at 1.3mg. Supplements usually start at 25-50mg.

Precautions:

B6 can interact with anti-epilepsy drugs, antibiotics, and drugs used for breathing problems.

High doses of B6 can cause neuropathy, a disorder of the nerves that can cause tingling and pain in the nerve endings.

Bromelain

Bromelain is an enzyme derived from pineapple. It is known to have anti-inflammatory properties and it is also helpful for the treatment of arthritis. It can be taken in tablet form and it is best taken on an empty stomach for better absorption.

Sources:

Bromelain is best taken as a supplement as there is not enough of the enzyme in pineapple for it to be effective when ingested that way.

Dosage:

For injuries, bromelain should be taken at 500mg a day and upwards.

Side Effects:

Precautions:

Bromelian should not be taken by pregnant women, by people with blood pressure problems or by patients with liver or kidney disease.

People on blood thinning drugs, antibiotics or sedatives should speak to a GP as bromelian may interact with these types of medication.

5) Glucosamine chondroitin sulphate

A study carried out by the Department of Orthopaedics and Trauma at Gaza University, Turkey, in 2011 and published in the PubMed Journal showed that rats fed on glucosamine chondroitin sulphate showed increased tendon strength, less inflammation and an increased rate of collagen formation. The researchers concluded that glucosamine helped to heal the tendon by reducing inflammation and stimulating collagen synthesis.

Side Effects:

Glucosamine is usually safe to take, but it can cause digestive upsets in some people.

Dosage:

This supplement is available in doses of up to 1500mg.

Precautions:

Glucosamine should not be taken without medical advice. Patients with diabetes should speak to their consultant before taking this supplement as it can adversely affect blood sugar control.

Patients with shellfish allergies should also be careful with this product, and people on blood thinning medications should speak to their doctor before taking glucosamine..

6) MSM

MSM is often taken by people with inflammatory joint conditions such as arthritis. However, MSM is also thought to be beneficial in tendon repair and MSM does play a role in collagen synthesis and aids in the production of collagen.

MSM is also believed to relieve pain.

Side Effects:

Some people report headaches and digestive upsets.

Precautions: There are no reported drug interactions, however, if you are being treated for a medical condition, so seek advice before supplementing.

7) Cissus

Cissus is a product popular with body builders. Cissus is an Indian remedy that is often used to help heal broken bones. However, the product is also thought to be beneficial for people with tendon problems.

Cissus is believed to aid in the regeneration of connective tissue and is thought to enable tendon injuries to heal quicker.

Side Effects:

Excessive sweating, digestive problems, and an increase in testosterone levels.

Precautions:

This supplement should not be taken by pregnant women. Too much of this product can cause drowsiness.

8) Manganese

Low levels of manganese can cause tendons to become more prone to injury and the mineral also contributes to the health of the tendons, ligaments and connective tissue. The recommended daily amount for adults aged 18 or over is 1.8mg. Some experts recommend a dosage of more than 30mg for aiding tendon health.

Sources:

Nuts, shellfish, seeds, soybeans.

Precautions:

Too much of this mineral can prove toxic and can also lower iron levels. Manganese also might interact with antipsychotic drugs, tetracycline antibiotics, anti-acids and other medications, so seek medical advice if you are thinking of supplementing with this mineral.

9) Amino Acids and Achilles Tendinopathy

Amino acids are the building blocks of protein. Amino acids play many different roles in helping our bodies to transmit nerves, aiding muscle function etc.

It is a good idea for people who put their bodies through a lot of grueling exercise regimes to supplement with amino acids as there is evidence to show that amino acids can help aid tissue growth and regeneration.

Specifically, supplementing with L Glutamine has been shown to help the Achilles tendon to heal quicker after an injury and studies have shown nitric oxide to be helpful in assisting the healing of an injured tendon.

10) Fish Oil

If there is inflammation present, then fish oil can help reduce this and can help to limit pain and swelling. Rather than taking fish oil as a supplement, it is better to eat oily fish as a regular part of your diet. However, if you are attempting to treat an injury, then capsules are a more effective way of supplementing the diet.

Sources:

Oily fish, fish oil supplements

Precautions:

People on blood thinning medication should not supplement with fish oil. Patients with blood clotting disorders should also avoid taking fish oil supplements.

11) Collagen

Our tendons are made up of 97% collagen, the fibrous proteins that help to form tendons and connective tissue. Supplementing with collagen capsules could help to speed up the healing of a damaged Achilles tendon.

Many brands of collagen capsules are available, and they are often sold as a beauty supplement to reduce the signs of aging and to improve the elasticity of the skin.

However, some people report side effects when supplementing with collagen as they can increase calcium levels in the body. Seek medical advice to see if taking collagen would be suitable in your case.

12) Growth Factors

A study published in the British Medical Journal suggests that growth factors could be useful in helping to speed up the healing of a damaged tendon. The study examined ways of introducing growth factors to the body via gene therapy. However, growth factor supplements can be bought from various body building stores, but as they can alter hormone levels, these types of supplements should not be taken without first getting some medical advice.

Chapter 8) Alternative Therapies

In an attempt to find relief from their symptoms, many people will start to look to alternative therapies. While many of these treatments can be beneficial in many ways, most of these treatments are designed to be complimentary and aren't meant to take the place of traditional medicine.

If you wish to try some of the alternative therapies available, then consult a doctor first. Moreover, when looking for alternative treatments, do your research carefully and follow these tips when looking for a practitioner:

Make sure that the person you are planning to see is fully qualified to treat you and your condition, Moreover, do some careful research first to find out the success rates of your treatment of choice.

1) Acupuncture

Acupuncture works by placing needles into the skin to release blocked energy or chi. It is thought that acupuncture works by triggering the release of pain-reducing opioids. It shouldn't be used by patients on blood thinning medications or by patients with a blood clotting disorder.

2) Tai Chi

If you are usually an active person, it can be frustrating to wait until you are able to return to your usual sports and activities. However, while you are waiting to get back into the sports you enjoy, there is an ideal opportunity to try something new.

Tai Chi is a slow paced form of exercise, but it can be every bit as challenging. Tai Chi is often described as meditation in motion, and the slow, smooth moves of Tai Chi certainly have a calming influence on the mind.

Tai Chi can also help to improve mobility, co-ordination and balance.

Chi Kung and Qi Qing also offers a gentle form of exercise to keep the mind and body active, and provide a good way of exercising while waiting to get back into normal exercise. The graceful movements of these types of meditative movements are a good alternative to stronger paced exercises and it would be a good idea to practice these forms of exercise more often once you do get back to your usual exercise routine in order to provide a contrast to your usual workouts and give the tendons and muscles a much needed rest as well as giving them an additional challenge.

3) Osteopathy

By using manipulation techniques, osteopaths believe that this technique can enable the body to heal itself. Osteopathy is often used for the treatment of sports injuries and can be used for Achilles tendonitis.

4) Alexander Technique

The Alexander Technique teaches patients how to reduce tension in their bodies. The technique helps people to walk better, stand better and to use their bodies in a safer, healthier way to avoid strain or stress.

People who use the Alexander Technique often say that, after years of pain and discomfort, they are able to walk freely and comfortably after practicing the technique.

5) Pilates

Pilates is essentially a mind-body technique. It involves very slow, small movements that encourage you to think about each muscle as you use it.

6) Chiropractic Therapy

A chiropractor is trained to help treat with the neuromusculoskeletal system. The emphasis is on releasing the joints, however, some patients with tendonitis might find this type of treatment useful for their condition as it will act to release tension throughout the body.

7) Trigger Point Therapy

Trigger Point Therapy is often used by therapists to reduce pain. The technique can be used to relieve all sorts of painful conditions including the pain caused by overuse injuries.

While many people find this an effective way of managing their pain, it should also be noted that with some people pressing on trigger points can make the pain worse. Unfortunately, the only way to determine if you will be one of the patients from this sore of treatment is by trying it.

Some people will experience a momentary soreness before finding relief, while others find that the pain takes longer to go away, but that this technique does work for them.

If this kind of treatment interests you, you'll find many books available on the subject.

8) The Elaine Petrone Method

The Elaine Petrone Method teaches the body to relax by releasing muscle tension and spasm throughout the body. While you are unlikely to find anyone teaching this method in the UK, a DVD is available. The DVD set includes the two small balls that you'll need to complete the exercises.

The method concentrates on helping the muscles to relax deeply, which in turn will reduce stress all over, but you can choose to concentrate on the lower leg muscles.

Chapter 9) Orthotics, Insoles, Splints and Aids

It wasn't that long ago that there was a limited range of products available for those with Achilles tendon injuries, however, there is now a huge selection of products to buy so it can be hard to determine which is the product for you. Sometimes it can just be a matter of trial and error and finding out what works best for you.

The first step in looking for orthotics or supports should be to talk to a sports therapist or a physiotherapist. They will be able to provide advice based on which product will be the most suitable for you personally, and this is a better option than buying products based on other people's reviews as what works for them might be entirely unsuitable for you.

It is also worth noting that if you have an on-going medical condition that contributes to your Achilles tendonitis your GP can refer you to a podiatrist at your local hospital. Sometimes the waiting list is long, but you'll get sound advice and you'll be able to get insoles or supports that are made especially for you and for your needs.

If this service isn't available from your local NHS or if the waiting list is too long and you don't want to wait, then there are plenty of services in the US and UK that can create orthotics especially for your needs. The best way to find a specialist company is to find one close to you, but you'll find many services online that can take a cast of your foot and produce something that is right for you. These products can be extremely expensive in some cases, but with some looking around you'll find many affordable options. This is an avenue well worth exploring especially if your injury is keeping you from doing the things you love or from enjoying your everyday life. You'll find a list of supplies at the back of this book.

1) McDavid Achilles Support

This product provides basic support to the Achilles area and also gives a mild compression to the Achilles to help control swelling and is useful for giving support when it comes to running and jumping.

The makers of the support recommend it for people who are prone to overuse injuries and for people with mild to moderate pain.

2) Spidertech Tape

SpiderTech Tape produce a product that is ready cut to give your Achilles and calf area the support it needs. The tape is made from kinesiology tape, a sports product that continues to grow in popularity and that is favoured by many top sports stars.

The tape is designed to enhance recovery time, reduce pain, and increase blood flow. As well as being used for Achilles tendons, it is also suitable for people with plantar fasciitis, shin splints or dropped arches. You can wear the product as you take part in swimming or running, and unlike some products, it won't limit the range of motion in your joints.

With this product, the work is done for you, so you don't have to worry about cutting the tape incorrectly. This is a great idea as strapping an injured foot incorrectly could cause the injury to become worse. However, the manufacturers advise that you get a therapist to apply the product for you, and the SpiderTech is designed for one use only, but can be worn for five days.

3) Heel Supports

Heel supports are often suggested to help reduce the Achilles pain and for calf strains, however, if you already have tight calves and if the tightness in your calves is contributing to your Achilles pain, then you might find this product is not right for you.

Heel lifts and supports can limit how much your calf has to stretch when you step. In some cases, this can make your calf tighter, and this could also make the problem with the Achilles worse.

4) Aircast Airsport Ankle Brace

This product is ideal for people who play a lot of sports such as tennis and badminton. It is an ankle support, rather than an Achilles, but if ankle weakness is a problem then this product can offer valuable support.

This product has been designed so that they are lightweight. Inside the support are two plastic stirrups that sit either side of the ankle to promote ankle stability. This ankle support offers a greater level of cushioning than some others on the market, but they are a little more expensive.

5) 1000 Mile Support Sock

This sock will provide compression to the foot and help with the rehabilitation of foot injuries. It can be used by people with Achilles tendinopathy, but it is also suitable for patients with plantar fasciitis, ankle sprains and other foot injuries.

As well as being used in the treatment of Achilles injuries, they can also be used for prevention by wearing them when taking part in sports or running.

6) Achilles Tendon Protector

The gel supports included in the Achilles tendon protector can give support to a recently injured tendon. Keeping the tendon protected should enhance the healing time and protect it from further injury.

The Achilles Tendon Protector is also designed for people with heel pain and Achilles bursitis.

7) Night Splints

Many people find that the symptoms of their tendonitis are worse in the morning. This is because our tendons tend to be tighter in the morning and also, the feet can go into a flexed position at night and this can pull on the Achilles.

A good night splint will hold your foot in the dorsiflexed position at night, making sure that your Achilles tendon stays extended all night long. If you have a foot drop due to a short Achilles, then this product might also be useful to you, but don't buy splints without first seeking medical advice.

There are a few negatives with splints that you should take into consideration. First of all, with some splints, the foot has a tendency to slide down the splint at night, leaving the foot pressed against the splint in a plantar flexed condition, and pulling on the Achilles.

Another problem is that they can rub against your skin, causing sore patches where the straps rest. This isn't so much of a problem with newer splints, but it is an issue you should be aware of especially if you are diabetic or if you have circulation problems. In some cases, you can get a piece a sheepskin to cover the strap with and this should help to protect your skin from rub marks.

If you don't want to wear the splints at night, you could wear them during the day when you are watching TV or when you know you won't need to be on your feet for a while. This isn't as effective as wearing the splint at night, but it will provide the Achilles with some additional rest.

As always, discuss with a sports therapist or a GP to help decide

101

which would be the best splint for you and don't rely upon other people's reviews.

8) Active Orthotics Night Splint

The Active Orthotics Night Splint comes with three straps that are padded out so they shouldn't catch against your skin as you sleep. The splint will give your Achilles a gentle stretch and help ensure that your tendon doesn't tighten up overnight.

These splints are best suited to people with Achilles tendonitis that has been caused by overuse. It is also useful for patients with plantar fasciitis.

9) ProCare Dorsiwedge Night Splint

This splint has been made for people with plantar fasciitis. However, as it holds the foot at a 90 degree angle, it can also be used to stretch the Achilles. The ProCare splint has much broader straps so they don't tend to rub against the skin so much and are more comfortable to wear during the night.

The splint also comes with a wedge insert, which can be used if the wearer wants to get a bit more of a stretch to the plantar fascia tendon.

10) Orthotics

If the problems with your Achilles are caused by a biomechanical problem, then it is likely that you'll be advised to consider wearing orthotics. These can be useful for shock absorption or in some cases of pronation; however, if you have excessive pronation then these types of insoles will not do much to correct this problem.

While some people swear by orthotics, some experts state that orthotics only serve to move the pain somewhere else. Orthotics doesn't address the underlying imbalances that cause the Achilles problem, and without addressing this, the pain isn't going to go anywhere.

Another thing to take into consideration is that wearing orthotics can initially make the pain worse for some people. When a new insert is worn in the shoe, it changes the way a person walks and changes the posture. Although these changes may be subtle, a change in the way someone walks can add an additional challenge to the muscles and tendons, forcing them to work harder or differently than they are used to, and this can cause further pain and increase the chances of overuse.

Orthotics are probably best for short term use while recovering from an injury, but should not be worn long term without addressing the issues that are causing the problem.

There are many different types of orthotics on the market and some of them have mixed reviews. This is generally because people have different needs and what will work for one person is not going to work for another.

In order to get an insole that is best for you, you'll need to see a sports therapist or a podiatrist, who can help make a pair of inserts suited to you. However, off the shelf orthotics can also work well for some people, and since they are affordably priced, they are something that are worth considering, even if they do only provide short term relief.

11) ¾ length insoles

These types of insoles will help with the alignment of the foot, and help reduce pronation to some degree. They are made for people with plantar fasciitis, but they are also suitable for Achilles problems.

If you have clawed toes or hammer toes then you might find these types of insoles better for you as they leave more space at the toe and they don't push your toes too close to the top of the shoe, which can cause friction.

12) Full length Orthotics

When wearing full length orthotics, care needs to be taken that they don't rub against the arch of the foot, making the inside of the arch sore. If you decide on these types of insoles and notice any kind of redness, then discontinue use.

Some full length orthotics come with additional arch support, however, you can also buy additional gel supports to attach them for a greater level of arch support if you wish. This can sometimes make the pain worse if your foot has to adapt to a new position, if this is the case for you, then remove the added inserts at the first hint of pain, as it won't get better the longer you leave the gel inserts in.

The items detailed below are just a small selection of what is available.

13) Fit Feet Full Length Orthotics

These full length orthotics have a medium density and they have a velour cover so they should feel comfortable against the skin. They reduce pronation, improve the alignment of the foot and help to reduce the pull and pressure on the Achilles tendon.

14) Heel Cups

Heel cups are often made of silicone so they are easy to clear and ideal if you intend to wear them a lot. They are also available very cheaply, so if you tend to wear them down quickly, then this isn't a problem.

The heel cups are designed for help with Achilles tendonitis, Achilles bursitis, plantar fasciitis and ankle pain. These cups are also good for people who walk about a lot or who spend a lot of time standing on their feet as they will act as shock absorbers, helping to take the impact out of the heel as you walk.

15) Wobble Board

If you have been away from your favourite exercise for a bit and have found that your balance has begun to suffer, then you should benefit from a wobble board. As well as improving balance, the wobble board will help to strengthen ankles that might have weakened after a period of inactivity and they are suggested for use once a person has reached the intermediate rehabilitation stage.

When it comes to managing your Achilles pain, you should also look at what else is going on within the muscles and tendons of the feet. For some people, the misalignment starts right at the toes and, gently loosening and lengthening clawed toes or hammer toes, can make a significant difference to the way you walk and the way you place your feet when you walk, all of which can have an impact on the Achilles tendon, contributing to the pain that you feel. Listed below are some of the options available for toe stretching.

16) Toe Stretchers

Toe Stretchers can be used to help the alignment of the toes, helping to stretch tight tendons and aiding mobility. While these are often intended for use by people with claw toes or tight muscles, they can also help restore the "bounce" to your walk, improve your posture, reduce pain; increasing the range of motion in your joins, aiding co-ordination and generally making walking easier.

17) Toe Alignment Socks

These socks offer a softer feel for people who might not like the feel of toe stretchers. Like the above product, these are designed to help lengthen the toes, thus improving mobility and reducing foot pain.

18) Yoga Toe Stretchers

Yoga toe stretchers will help to realign the toes and realign the structure of the feet. They can also aid circulation and posture and reduce the pain in your feet when you walk. If your toes are too clawed, then you might find these a little uncomfortable to wear, but they don't cost a lot to buy and they are worth trying if you are looking to improve the overall mobility of your feet.

19) Walking Cast Boot

If your case of Achilles tendonitis is severe then your consultant might suggest casting your foot to allow the tendon time to heal. If you are usually an active person, then this is a suggestion you might not be comfortable with.

Being in a cast often means that the wearer loses some muscle and it takes some time to regain mobility and strength afterwards. There is a viable alternative, which is to wear an Achilles tendon walking boot or walking cast.

20) DonJoy Walkabout Plastic Walker

This walking cast is designed for ankle injuries, fractures and stress fractures, but can also be used to help rest an overworked Achilles tendon. The cast allows a patient to walk around as they would normally, but without the stress or strain on the healing tendons.

The cast can be used as part of rehabilitation and can enhance healing time. When not wearing the cast, the patient can try some gentle stretching to maintain range of motion and to ensure that the Achilles tendon doesn't tighten up further.

There are also casts available that will use gentle compression to help reduce swelling. This might be useful to patients who have developed swelling in and around the ankle as a result of their Achilles injury.

21) Massage

Massage plays an important part in helping to keep muscles supple and can help reduce the tension around muscles, therefore releasing the strain from tendons. If you are extremely active or if your favourite sporting activity involves a lot of repetition, you will probably find that stretching on its own isn't enough, and you could benefit from a regular sports massage.

If you don't want to go to the expense of a regular appointment with a sports therapist then you could try massaging your lower leg area and ankles yourself using a massage lotion designed to help relax the muscles after exercise. There are also many books and DVDs on the subject of massage therapy, which are worth investing in to learn a few beneficial massage techniques.

Massage is best used before beginning to exercise to encourage circulation and warm up the muscles and again after your exercise session. The stronger your muscles get, the tighter they will be, so a massage after exercising will help return your muscles to their relaxed state.

Moreover, the circulation to the Achilles tendon is slow, which might be one of the reasons why it is so slow to heal. Massage can help increase circulation, which may aid healing.

22) Akileline Sports Cold Cream

This massage cream has been formulated to help increase circulation. The cream also has a cooling effect, which should help if you have the burning pain that comes with some Achilles injuries.

The products listed in this chapter are not personal endorsements or recommendations. They merely give an idea of the products out there. With some proper research, you'll find hundreds of similar products available.

Some of the products are designed to reduce pronation, while others are designed to help the Achilles heel, reduce swelling, and improve balance and healing times. However, none of these items should be bought without getting advice on which ones are best suited to you.

23) Hot and Cold Therapy Pack

These versatile packs can be frozen or warmed up according to your needs. With some people, they find that cold can make the pain worse, while others find that warmth works better for them. If you choose to freeze the pack, then don't hold it directly against the skin and only use for a maximum of twenty minutes.

The same applies if you choose to heat the pack. Don't hold it directly against the skin because of the chance that it could burn.

24) Thermoactive Ankle Support

The Thermoactive Ankle Support has been created for people with Achilles Tendonitis, Achilles bursitis, plantar fasciitis, ankle pain and inflammation. Unlike the conventional ankle wraps, this will cover the entire of your ankle region and provide compression to the injured area.

The manufacturers of the product advise customers to consult their doctor before using the wrap to ensure it is suitable for them.

25) Insolia

Insolia arch supports are much thinner and smaller than traditional insoles and are designed for people who wear high heels, which means that their foot is held in a plantar flexed position, meaning it will put stress on the tendon.

These supports are designed to provide a superior level of support for the foot while it is in the planter flexed position. It will also take away the pressure on the balls of the feet and reduce lower back pain and leg pain.

If you tend to walk plantar flexed, so your toes go down before your heels, then you might find that this type of support is more suited to you.

Chapter 10) Footwear

Proper footwear can play a crucial part in preventing Achilles tendonitis, however, if you have already developed a tendon problem then it is a matter of finding a pair of shoes that won't make the problem worse.

Finding comfortable footwear when you have Achilles tendonitis can prove to be a bit of a challenge. If there is swelling, then this can make it uncomfortable to wear your normal shoes, and trying to break in new shoes while dealing with an Achilles injury isn't the best idea as your foot has to adjust to a different way of being held, and this can trigger more pain and imbalances.

You'll need to look for something that is supportive, but you won't want something that is too rigid, as holding the injured foot in one position will only add to the discomfort.

Trainers can also cause Achilles tendon problems and it is believed that some of the trainers designed for running can actually contribute to Achilles tendonitis and other problems with the Achilles.

Comfort rite make a range of shoes that are designed to reduce foot pain. As well as providing shock absorption, the shoes help to control excessive pronation and they are suitable for people with flat feet or ankle pain.

Orthofeet make shoes that have a customised orthotic already included as well as an ergonomic sole for added comfort. This range of footwear is especially helpful for people with heel pain, but they are also good for people with pronation, ankle and arch pain and for people with flat feet.

New Balance produce a range of trainers designed to give comfort for people who do a lot of walking and running. The shoes offer motion control, as well as providing stability to the foot and cushioning. The trainers are designed for people with Achilles tendonitis, heal pain and plantar fasciitis.

Darco manufacture a range of shoes for diabetics. However, the shoes are also suitable for people with heal pain, pronation and flat feet.

Aetex shoes are biomechanically designed to help reduce foot pain. They also help to prevent pain by reducing the level of stress put on the foot and are suitable for a large range of foot problems including tendonitis.

Finn Comfort has created a range of shoes and sandals designed for walking. The shoes offer a high level of orthopaedic support and are ergonomically designed for maximum comfort. The foot beds contained within the shoe have been designed to fit a customised orthotic, providing maximum support for the wearer.

Webster's supply a range of shoes for men and women that are designed to help provide comfort for people with Achilles tendonitis. They also provide insoles, heel pads, bespoke insole and bespoke shoes.

http://webstershoes.co.uk/orthopaedic-shoes/achillestendonitis-160.shtml

For customers based in the United States, Murray's Shoes supply orthopaedic shoes that are designed to give additional comfort for people suffering from Achilles tendonitis, pronation, flat feet and other foot problems.

Simply Feet has orthotic footwear that already comes complete with an Aided Motion System ™ to improve that gait and to improve ease of movement.

Custom Orthotics

As explained earlier, it is best to have a pair of orthotics that has been designed specifically for you. If you find that this isn't something that is assessable to you, then you'll have to consider going private. Listed below are details of some companies based in the US or the UK, that can work with you to ensure that you get a pair of orthotics that are suitable for your needs.

Orthodynamics

Orthodynamics provide custom foot braces and insoles. These are available by prescription only. The braces will help reduce the severe pronation that can lead to Achilles tendon problems and will also offer support to the ankles.

Pedag USA

Pedag USA offers a range of inserts and orthotics that are designed to reduce pronation when you walk. They are also suitable for people with flat feet or Pes Planus. These are all conditions that will cause excessive stress to the Achilles tendon and plantar fasciitis when you walk.

Orthotics Online

Orthotics Online offer a free consultation. In order to create a pair of custom orthotics, patients must first undergo a biomechanical assessment and a computerised gait analysis. Measurements will also be taken of the foot and a cast created. Orthotics are created for a wide range of foot problems including Achilles tendonitis and pronation.

http://www.orthotics-online.co.uk/foot-problems.html

Orthotics

Orthotics Online

The company sells a range of orthotics and can also provide custom orthotics to add additional support for the heel and ankle. They also offer gait analysis to get a better idea of how an individual's foot is functioning, and provide custom made orthotics to help address the problem.

They also supply arch supports, heel lifts, heel cups and a range of other foot care products.

http://orthotics-online.co.uk/store/index.php?main_page=product_info&cPath=5&products_id=11

Sports Orthotics

If activity is the main trigger area for your tendonitis, then Sports Orthotics supply a range of products designed to readdress issues such as pronation etc.

The range of orthotics is available for purchase online, however, if you live in Scotland and live near enough to the clinic then they offer free biomechanical assessments so that they can provide a custom made orthotic designed to meet the customer's needs.

http://www.sportorthotics.co.uk/index.html

Foot Technology

Foot Technology supply a large range of orthotics that are designed to help address the many problems that can contribute to Achilles tendonitis such as high arches, flat feet, pronation etc.

They supply a line of orthotics suitable for people with Achilles tendonitis.

http://www.foottechnology.co.uk/ankle_pain.html

London Orthotics Consultancy

The London Orthotics Consultancy is a professional company offering specialist orthoses, braces and supports for joint stabilisation, foot pain, mobility issues, and to reduce the chance of injury.

They provide products for both adults and children and can assess, cast, design and create a custom made orthotic for clients. As well as providing these services to people in the London area, they also have clinics in Bristol and Leicester.

http://londonorthotics.co.uk/orthotics/?gclid=CMHT4KHxxbkCF YPHtAodP3oAWg

Chapter 11) Blogs and Forums

It can be useful to read other people's accounts of how they deal with their own Achilles injury. People will often discover things that work for them – often quite by accident. Finding suggestions that you might not have thought of can help relieve discomfort, at least to a degree. It is also helpful to know that you are not on your own and that there are plenty of people out there who have found ways of managing their condition, or in some cases have undergone successful surgery and got relief in that way.

While you should take into consideration that their solutions might not work for you, when it comes to treating a condition that is difficult to target, it's is always good to gain as much information as you can.

These blogs are just some of the blogs available; you'll find a huge list of Achilles blogs on the Internet. There are plenty of people sharing their experiences, and who knows, they might provide just the answer you are looking for.

Achillesblog.com

This helpful blog is a community that brings people together who are experiencing Achilles problems. You'll find information on all aspects of Achilles injuries, including tendonitis, rupture and Achilles tears.

When visiting the site you'll notice the many accounts by users detailed with their recoveries, explaining how they cope with pain, and asking general information. This is all very sound advice and can help provide some of the information you'll need to treat your own condition.

There are also many resources on this site including the latest information about studies, choosing a doctor and tips for finding a therapist.

http://achillesblog.com/

Achilles Tendon Drama

This entertaining blog is almost certain to make you feel better. It details the blog owner's experience of an Achilles rupture and the surgery that followed, but it is also about tendonitis and Achilles tears.

The process of surgery and the on-going rehabilitation will give someone with an Achilles rupture at least some idea of what to expect.

http://achillestendondrama.blogspot.co.uk/

My Ruptured Tendon

As well as detailing their recovery from an Achilles injury, this blog also reviews some useful products that people might find helpful as they continue their rehabilitation.

http://myrupturedtendon.blogspot.co.uk/

Achilles Tendon Rupture – Conservative Treatment

Making the decision to undergo surgery can be a difficult one, however, readers of this blog can be assured that they are not the only one facing this choice and visitors can read one person's account of how they managed to recover from an Achilles rupture without the need for surgery.

This is a great blog for anyone wrestling with this decision, and wanting to avoid having surgery.

http://achillestendonruptureconservative.blogspot.co.uk/

FORUMS

There are many sports forums online that can provide invaluable advice for people who are suffering from an Achilles injury. As an Achilles injury is such a common sports injury, there are plenty of people out there who have their own experiences to tell and are happy to share them.

It is possible to find ideas and solutions to aid your Achilles injury that you might never have thought of by yourself and it is also worth learning from other people's experiences, and from someone who has suffered the same problem.

The people on the forums are usually extremely helpful and they are only too glad to give advice on a range of subjects from finding the right trainers to rehabilitation following an injury.

Forums can also serve as a reminder that, although painful and debilitating, people do find ways of managing their Achilles problems, and are able to get back into doing the sports they love.

Fitness and Lifestyle.co.uk

As well as general discussions on fitness and wellbeing, there are also questions on rehabilitation that are useful for those recovering from a sports injury. If you have a question, just sign up and log in to get help, there is sure to be someone who can give some advice.

http://www.fitnessandlifestyle.co.uk/forum/10-general-discussion/

Bodybuilding.com

The main focus of the forum is nutrition and exercise, however, for anyone recovering from injury and who might have lost some muscle during the recovery phase, there is plenty of sound advice on rebuilding muscles and taking the correct supplements. There is also information on building calf muscle, stretching and using proper form, which is vital when it comes to avoiding injury.

http://forum.bodybuilding.com/forumdisplay.php?f=1

Shape Fit.com

Shapefit.com is full of helpful advice on training, yoga, diet, product reviews and there are a number of discussions about Achilles tendon surgery, injuries etc.

http://www.shapefit.com/forum/

John Stone Fitness.com

The forum has a category dedicated to injury issues. There are many discussions on Achilles injury, Achilles soreness and building calf muscles.
http://forums.johnstonefitness.com/search.php?searchid=2221843

Body Active Nation

The forum has a category dedicated to sports injury and prevention. There are discussions on tight Achilles, as well as other overuse injuries, and members are free to post their own questions if they are looking for advice.

http://www.bodyactive-nation.co.uk/forum

Chapter 12) Research

Recent research has led to a better understanding of Achilles tendonitis/tendinopathy and in the future it will hopefully lead to more treatments becoming available to patients. As doctors and scientists begin to understand more about the Achilles tendon, it enables them to look at new ways of managing the complex issues of Achilles tendonitis and other Achilles problems.

Although much of this research won't offer new treatments in the near future, anyone copying with this kind of problem will eventually have more options available to them when this type of injury occurs.

This chapter details some of the latest research, and some of the newer approaches to treating tendon problems.

Detecting Achilles Tendon Damage Early

Anyone with an Achilles injury should know how important it is to get the condition diagnosed and treated as soon as possible, and it could soon become much easier to get an early diagnosis, thus ensuring that the tendon is treated sooner rather than later.

According to a 2012 study by the Medical University of Vienna, Achilles tendon damage is possible to diagnose in its early stages by using sodium imaging and T2 mapping.

The researchers suggest that a high sodium level is indicative of potential problems to come with the Achilles tendon. T2 mapping is another way of detecting possible problems with the Achilles. T2 is an MR Parameter. Mapping the T2 levels makes it possible to detect any changes to the tendon that could later turn to damage.

Treatment of Flat Feet

Flat feet are a known cause of Achilles tendonitis and other foot problems, but there could be hope on the horizon for adults who have acquired this condition.

A study by the University of East Anglia states that flat feet is a condition commonly experienced in women over the age of forty. The problem is caused by the stretching of the tibialis posterior tendon - the tendon which acts like a sling for the arch and stabilises it. This condition can be more common in people with diabetes, who are obese, or who have high blood pressure.

The researchers found that in these cases there is an increased level of proteolytic enzymes, and these enzymes can break down the posterior tendon, causing it to weaken and the arch to flatten.

Researchers say that this discovery could possibly lead to new drug treatments that would target these enzymes, thus bringing relief to people with flat feet or people with Achilles tendonitis. However, the researchers advise that a drug therapy such as this is at least a decade away.

New Discovery Uncovers Clues to Tendon Injury

Researchers from Queen Mary, University of London, have discovered a vital component called the interfascicular matrix that could help find new treatments for Achilles tendon injuries.

The interfascicular matrix is responsible for binding the fascicles of the tendon together, and researchers think that an alteration in this component could lead the way to Achilles injuries.

Doctors believe that it could be possible to alter the interfascicular matrix, and if they are able to achieve this, it could lead to the development of diagnostic tests to discover if some people are more prone to tendon injuries and it could also lead to new treatments for overuse injuries.

Curcumin for Tendonitis

A study published by The University of Nottingham and Ludwig Maximilians University in Munich, shows that a well-known curry spice could be a useful aid in the treatment of Achilles tendonitis.

Scientists say that curcumin could help to reduce the mechanisms that trigger the inflammation that then triggers some Achilles tendon disorders.

During the research, the doctors discovered that curcumin could switch off a compound and prevent it from causing more inflammation.

Achilles tendons don't heal themselves

Anyone with an Achilles injury will know what a long journey it is before the tendon will start to heal. Poor circulation and blood flow to the tendon is one reason for the slow rate of healing, however, research published in 2013 sheds further light on the matter.

Research published in the Federation of American Societies for Experimental Biology shows that the Achilles tendon does not repair itself.

Katja Heinemeier, Ph.D., a researcher involved in the work from the Institute of Sport Medicine and Center for Healthy Aging at the University of Copenhagen in Denmark, conducted the research by using the nuclear fallout from World War II bomb tests and the carbon-14 peaks that resulted.

As part of the study, researchers examined the tendons of people

121

who lived through the carbon peaks and found that high levels of carbon still existed in the tendons.

The researchers believe that the reason the carbon still existed in the tendons was because the tendon does not renew itself . It is hoped the research will lead to new treatments for tendon problems.

Chapter 13) Clinics

If you don't want to wait for treatment for your Achilles injury then going to a private clinic is the quickest option. Most people should have a private hospital like the Nuffield near enough to them. If they don't then that will mean travelling to one of the specialists in the UK.

The clinics listed below are not recommendations, they just offer an example of some of the specialist services available to people with Achilles problems.

The Sports Injury Clinic

The Sports Injury Clinic has advice on more than 350 different sports injuries. There is plenty of information on Achilles injuries and there is a wealth of information on finding therapists and rehabilitation exercises, as well as suggested treatments and therapies.

http://www.sportsinjuryclinic.net/rehabilitation-exercises/lower-leg-ankle-exercises

Pure Sports Medicine

Based in London, Pure Sports Medicine offers a range of treatments for Achilles tendonitis. Patients attending the clinic will be given an ultrasound scan so their injury can be assessed; regular tendon clinics are held.

The clinic also offers PRP injections, which have been shown to be effective in the treatment of tendonitis.

http://www.puresportsmed.com/

Premier Foot and Ankle Clinic

The Premier Foot and Ankle Clinic is based in London and offers specialist treatment for Achilles tendon problems. As well as offering surgery, the clinic can also provide orthotics and insoles. They also provide treatment for heel pain and for a range of other foot complaints.

http://www.premierfootandankleclinic.com/www.premierfootandankleclinic.coms/info.php?p=8

Foot and Ankle Clinic

The Foot and Ankle Clinic is based in Surrey and they offer treatment and surgical techniques for foot problems, including Achilles tendonitis. Their specialists ensure that they are up-to-date with all of the latest methods so patients can be assured that they can access the latest in new techniques.

http://www.footandankleclinic.co.uk/foot-and-ankle-specialists/

The Hampshire Foot and Ankle Clinic

The clinic offers specialist care for foot and ankle problems. Among the treatments offered are shockwave therapy, physiotherapy and podiatry.

http://www.foot-ankle.co.uk/content/homepage/

American Orthopaedic Foot and Ankle Surgery Society

For those based in the United States, the American Orthopaedic Foot and Ankle Surgery Society has a wealth of resources to help.

The site is full of resources for people with foot and ankle problems.

You will also find a list of surgeons so it is easy to find a specialist that can help with your condition.

http://www.aofas.org/footcaremd/Pages/footcaremd.aspx

Windsor Foot and Ankle Clinic

The clinic offers a range of services from physiotherapy to insoles designed to help address any biomechanical issues. They can help with Achilles problems, sports injuries, ankle pain, and an array of other foot conditions.

http://www.windsorfoot.com/

Exeter Foot and Ankle Clinic

For those living in the south West, the Exeter Foot and Ankle clinic can offer a range of diagnostic services and treatments for patients with ankle and foot pain.

They treat tendon problems and sports related injuries. The clinic will arrange a consultation first so that they can discuss how best they can help.

http://www.exeterfootandankle.com/foot-and-ankle-problems.html

Lancashire Foot and Ankle Clinic

The clinic offers a vast range of services for those suffering with foot problems. They can also help in the case of Achilles ruptures. Appointments can be booked online.

http://www.lancashirefootclinic.co.uk/foot-ankle-lancashire-foot-ankle-clinic.html

Chapter 14) Prevention

Everyone is familiar with the saying that "prevention is better than cure" and this is also true of Achilles tendonitis. Once the Achilles has become damaged it takes a long time to repair itself – sometimes months or even years – and once a problem with the tendon develops it becomes more susceptible to injury.

Fortunately, such problems are largely avoidable and can be prevented if proper care is taken. Here are some tips to help prevent Achilles tendonitis.

Achilles tendonitis is common in runners. If running is your favourite activity, then ensure you protect the Achilles by wearing adequate footwear and by wearing orthotics if necessary.

A good sportswear store will be able to advise you on the best pair of trainers for your particular sport and can usually give advice on orthotics as well.

If the way you move is causing an unnecessary strain on the Achilles then go for a gait analysis. A gait analysis will provide detail on how the foot functions when in motion and a custom pair of orthotics can be designed specifically for your needs.

Rest

It can be tempting to work out every day and some people feel guilty if they don't exercise. However, your tendons need some time off from the strain of exercise, especially if you are placing demands on the tendons that they just can't cope with.

Take at least one day off from training a week and make it a day

126

when you stretch, do yoga or have a massage to help release any tension that might have accumulated in your muscles.

Work at your own pace

When competing with others or attending a class, it is too easy to think that you have to outdo someone else or keep up with the next person. However, we are all different and some of us just can't move as quickly as others, and some of us aren't as agile. Moreover, some people are just more prone to tendon problems. Don't risk an injury by pushing yourself too far and work at your own pace.

Stretch

If you don't already include a stretch routine as part of your regular workout, now is the time to introduce one. Stretching helps to elongate muscles that contract during exercise so it is important to ensure your muscles and tendons are returned to their relaxed position after exercising. Missing the occasional stretch after exercising is unlikely to do any harm, however, regular exercising without balancing it out with a stretch routine will inevitably lead to tight muscles, which will in turn lead to conditions such as tendinopathy.

Chapter 15) Sources

http://www.ncbi.nlm.nih.gov/pubmed/16463375

Eccentric Training in Achilles Tendinopathy: Is it harmful to the tendon?

http://www.ncbi.nlm.nih.gov/pmc/articles/PMC2465326/
eccentric training

Posterior Tibial Tendon Dysfunction: More prevalent in Women

http://www.aaos.org/news/aaosnow/mar09/research7.asp

Long-term use of high heeled shoe alters the neuromechanics of human walking

http://www.ncbi.nlm.nih.gov/pubmed/22241055

http://www.newswise.com/articles/pretty-shoes-can-lead-to-ugly-foot-problems-for-women

http://www.prnewswire.com/news-releases/achilles-tendon-injuries-more-likely-in-male-weekend-warriors-than-others-204287491.html

Achilles Tendon Injury Statistics

http://www.fleetfeetsyracuse.com/news/sos-injury-prevention-treatment-blog-achilles-tendon-injuries

Insertional Achilles Tendonitis

http://www.aofas.org/footcaremd/conditions/ailments-of-the-ankle/Pages/Insertional-Achilles-Tendinitis.aspx

http://www.firstaid4sport.co.uk/Achilles-Bursitis-Ainjury_achillesbursitis/

http://phys.org/news161516132.html

http://orthoinfo.aaos.org/topic.cfm?topic=a00147

http://www.podiatrytoday.com/understanding-how-the-achilles-tendon-affects-plantar-pressure

High-dose vitamin C supplementation accelerates the Achilles tendon healing in healthy rats

http://www.ncbi.nlm.nih.gov/pubmed/18309503

Effect of Glucosamine chondroitin sulphate on repaired tentotomized rat Achilles tendons

http://www.ncbi.nlm.nih.gov/pubmed/21762066

Achilles Tendon Injuries in Athletes

http://www.ncbi.nlm.nih.gov/pubmed/7809555

Nitric Acid

http://inotekcorp.com/publications/pdf/ipcpub44.pdf

Growth factors:

http://bjsm.bmj.com/content/36/5/315.full

Women and Achilles problems:

http://www.biomedcentral.com/1471-2474/11/41

Estrogen and Achilles problems

http://www.footlogic.com/pdf/etiologic-factors-associated-with-symptomatic-achilles-tendinopathy.pdf

New methods enable the early detection of Achilles tendon damage:

http://www.alphagalileo.org/ViewItem.aspx?ItemId=116660&CultureCode=en

First step towards treatment of painful flat feet

http://www.alphagalileo.org/ViewItem.aspx?ItemId=115860&CultureCode=en

Scientists discover new clues explaining tendon injury

http://www.eurekalert.org/pub_releases/2012-07/qmuo-sdn070312.php

Curry spice could offer treatment hope for tendonitis

http://www.eurekalert.org/pub_releases/2011-08/uon-csc080911.php

Fallout from Nuclear Testing Shows Achilles cannot Heal itself

http://www.eurekalert.org/pub_releases/2013-02/foas-ffn021213.php

Further reading

Treat your own Achilles Tendonitis by Johnson, Jim

Achilles Healing: Achilles Tendonitis Relief and Prevention in Four Easy Steps by Hafner, Patrick

Fixing Your Feet by VonHof, John

Yoga for Sports by Christensen, Alice

Sport and Remedial Massage by Cash, Mel

The BMA Guide to Sports Injuries

Sports Rehabilitation and Injury prevention by Comfort, Paul

DVDs

Restorative Exercises for Foot Pain

Yoga for Athletes

Athletes Guide to Yoga

Yoga Conditioning for Athletes

Yoga for Runners

Power Yoga for Runners

Glossary

Cortisol: The hormone released by the adrenal glands when the body is under stress

Gait: The way a person moves

Gait Analysis: An assessment of the way a person moves

Pronation: The inward roll of the foot

Evert: The way the foot points outwards when walking

Posterior tibial tendon dysfunction: An inflammation of the tendon that runs into the inside of the ankle; the tendon supports the arch of the foot.

Soleus: The muscle in the back part of the lower leg

NSAIDS: Non-steroidal Anti-inflammatory drug

Opioids: A drug that acts like morphine

Growth Factors: A protein molecule

Biomechanics: How the tendons, muscles etc., work together in the human body

Plantar fasciitis: An inflammation of the plantar tendon, which runs from the bottom of the foot all the way along to the big toe.

Hammer Toes: A contracted toe

Orthotics/ Orthoses: A range of products that help to correct various biotechnical problems

AFO: Ankle Foot Orthotic

Tendinopathy: A degeneration of the tendon

Kinesiology tape: A tape made from elastic that is used to support the joints and tendons after injury

Index

CPSIA information can be obtained
at www.ICGtesting.com
Printed in the USA
BVHW03s0319110518
515768BV00008B/145/P